SEXUAL SECRETS

• A LOVER'S GUIDE TO SEXUAL ECSTASY •

MEDIAPRESS

Sexual Enrichment Series™

DEDICATED TO SAFE HEALTHY SEX

Some of the photographs in this book depict sexual activity that could be unsafe if practiced without a condom with a partner infected with a sexually transmitted disease (including AIDS and HIV). We support the right of all adults to any consensual sexual activity. However, we urge anyone at the slightest risk to practice the safest sex possible. If you have questions about safe sex, contact your local health department.

IMPORTANT: PLEASE READ

Some of the positions shown in this publication require above average physical strength, more than the average man or woman can sustain for the normal length of intercourse. Do not strain your body beyond its capacity. Should any strain occur, consult a medical professional immediately. Be cautious about the angle of entry for the penis. An awkward thrusting position can be dangerous, as the penis can sustain damage if it is excessively bent.

SEXUAL SECRETS
A LOVER'S GUIDE TO SEXUAL ECSTASY
Copyright © 1987, 1992 MEDIA PRESS
P.O. Box 4326, Chatsworth, CA 91311

ISBN 0–917181–30–1

10 9 8 7 6 5   Cover photograph by Mark Efford   Printed in U.S.A.

CONTENTS

INTRODUCTION

Sexual Secrets: A Lover's Guide to Sexual Ecstasy is just that–a guide. It needn't be read from cover to cover like a work of fiction, although you may choose to do so. Rather, it is more like a reference book that you can open to any chapter that interests you and find what you're looking for.

It has been observed on many occasions—often when an instant philosophical justification is needed to explain a lapse in judgment—that variety is the spice of life. This is commonly interpreted to mean that a variety of *partners* is necessary to maintain sexual interest. Variety can be obtained not only from numerous partners, but also from a variety of settings,

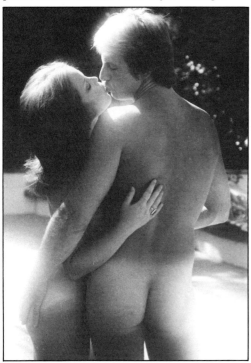

positions, and fantasies with the *same* partner. Thus, sharing this book with a caring, sexually compatible partner is the ideal situation.

The term "positions manual" sounds like something one would find in a time capsule from the 1950s. It recalls little Baby Boomers going through their fathers' dresser drawers looking for photos of naked women (and praying that sex would someday be legalized in the Midwest). Those days are gone, and naked women—and men—can be seen in coffee table

magazines and on television (although sex is still illegal in several Midwestern states). But though we have all seen the human form undraped on countless occasions, most of us still find it sufficiently mysterious, exciting, and erotic to devote considerable energy to its pursuit. Sex is still right up there on the Survival Top Ten List just below food and video.

Whereas nudity and sexual opportunity are no longer in short supply, quality sexual activity—or at least *knowledgeable* sexual activity—often is. Consider this: what is sex education? One would think that whatever it was, it would have something to do with education about sex. But no, it's merely information

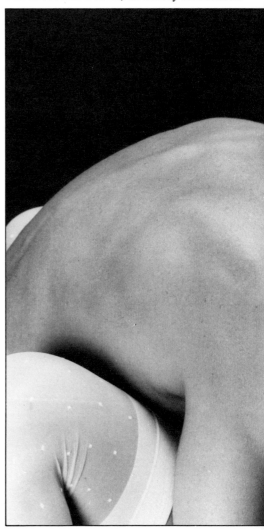

about contraception and a little basic anatomy. It seems part of the human condition that we are doomed to remain ignorant about the things that affect us most. Each of us, regardless of race, sex, status, or education, is born and must die. However, even in the age of high tech and quantum physics, much of what we know about birth and death is still mystical in nature, full of conjecture, superstition, fear, and ignorance.

The same can be said of our sparse knowledge of sex. Young men and women have nowhere to go to learn about sex—only how not to make a baby. In some parts of the world, the practice of female circumcision—cutting out the clitoris—is still in vogue. Many men—and

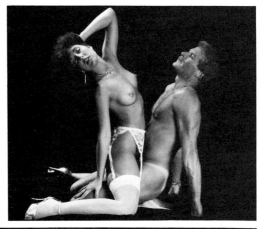

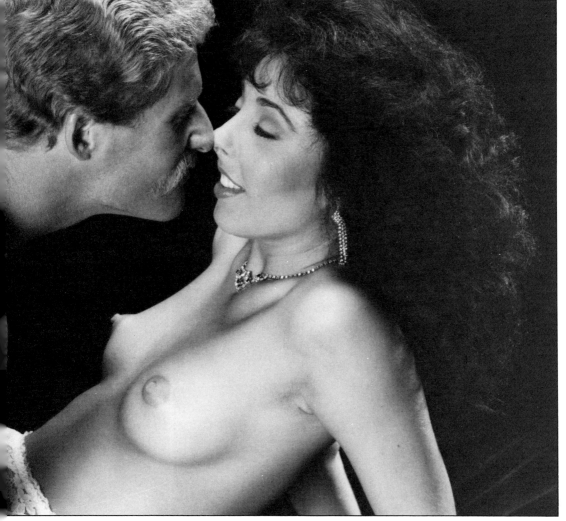

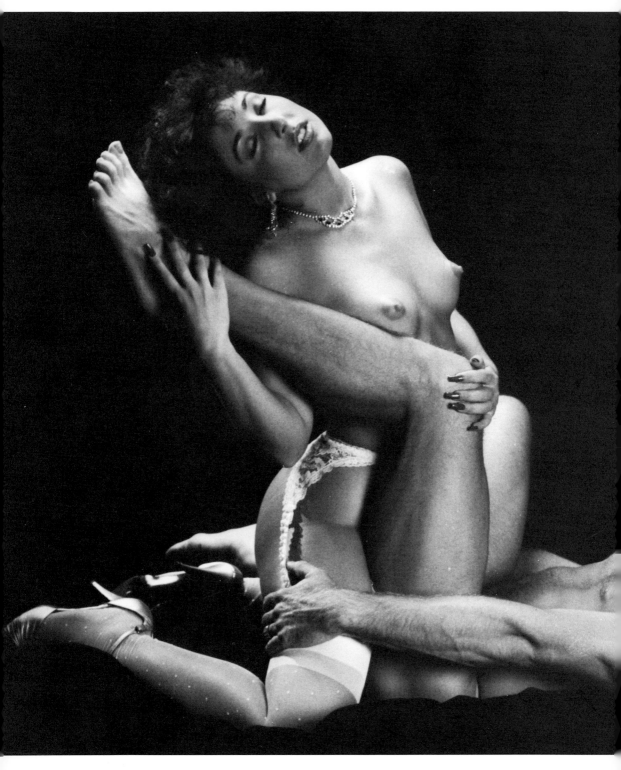

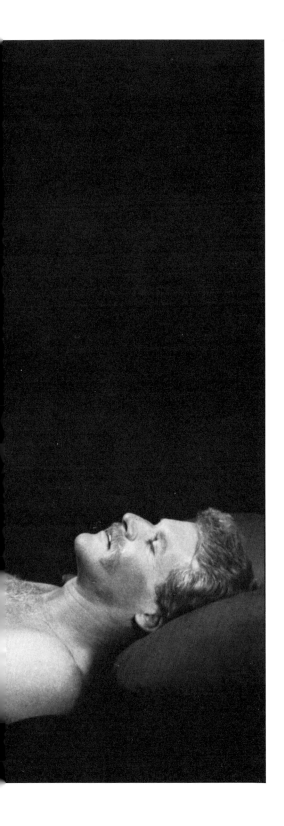

even some women—still need a road map in order to find the clitoris.

We wouldn't expect someone who didn't know how to turn on a computer to do word processing, yet we expect people to become skillful lovers on instinct alone. The human body is so much more sophisticated—and beautifully so—than a computer. Go to a bookstore sometime and see how many books you can find on computers and how many books on how to make love. You'll find hundreds of books on romance, sex, and nudity, but a paltry few on how to make love. Many bookstores even refuse to carry such material because of its "explicit nature"—the term implying that there is something "obscene" about such material. Why a bookstore or television network can proudly display visions of death, murder, rape, beating, mutilation, and catastrophe and, just as proudly, refuse to depict human beings without their clothes on, or while making love, is a great and sad human mystery, and beyond the scope of this book.

Whether there has or has not been an outright conspiracy to keep human beings in the dark about sex, the effect is the same: people still know very little about their own bodies or their partners' bodies. Perhaps this book will play a small part in changing that.

DIFFERENT STROKES . . .
Experimenting with different positions is not only enjoyable, it's also logical. Many men have had the experience of making love to a woman and noticing that a certain position provides his partner and/or himself with intense sensation. Soon afterward, the same man might try the same position with another woman and get little, if any, of the same sensation or response.

The reason for this is simple, though not always recognized. Not all bodies are alike. They come in different sizes and shapes. I have a friend who is nearly seven feet tall. He was dating a woman who was barely over five feet in high heels. He had to change his lovemaking techniques considerably in order to maximize their mutual pleasure. However, after making those adjustments—and they came through trial and error—their sexual relationship soared.

Another friend, Edward H., told me of an experience he had shortly after his wife gave

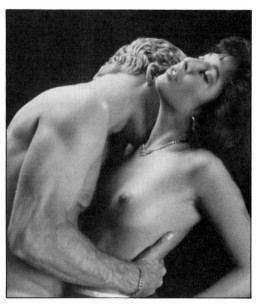

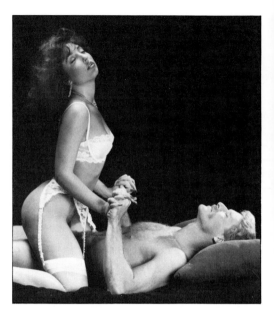

birth to their first child. Previously he and his wife had enjoyed what my friend called a "superior" sexual relationship. On one occasion he volunteered the observation that they fit together sexually "like a hand in a velvet glove."

After the birth of their child, however, this "fit" changed drastically. While lamenting his troubles to a friend one night, the friend suggested that Edward take a look at a book the friend had on sexual positions. Edward, distraught and despondent, at first waved off the idea. But eventually he relented.

Although he didn't immediately try the different positions he read about in the book, Edward gradually began to experiment with a slightly different sexual repertoire. Two immediate benefits resulted. First, his wife was excited by the variety that the new positions brought to the couple's sex life. Second, and more important, the husband discovered that there were several positions, particularly positions that called for him to enter his wife from behind, that brought back the old feelings of fitting hand-in-glove.

What this means is that while men and women generally fit together well, size variations do exist, and some positions accommodate these variations better than others.

The only requirements are a willing partner and a little imagination (or at least an imaginative

and understandable manual). Not to take advantage of what nature has to offer is a little like walking into the best clothing store in town, with an unlimited budget, and trying on only one suit of clothes. It's *your* sex life—your's and your partner's. Why not take advantage of as many possibilities as you can?

"But I've tried all those exotic positions," you say. Chances are, you haven't really tried them all. And what have you got to lose anyhow? So you try ten positions, and you hate nine of them. All that means is that you and your lover have one new position that you wouldn't have known about otherwise that you can use to give each other pleasure for the rest of your lives.

ATTITUDE
To say that attitude in sexual relations is everything may be overstating the case, but not by much.

Do you remember the first time you made love with someone you subsequently developed a relationship with? Do you remember how "hot" and passionate those first lovemaking sessions were? Even though sex may still be quite enjoyable with that person, if you're like most people, your sexual relations have probably cooled with time and familiarity. Ask most people about this phenomenon and they'll tell you that's just the way it is, that there's no way around sexual interest waning with the passing of time. Is it any wonder, then, that sexually active people leave an endless trail of wet-sheeted beds in their wake, as they go through an endless number of not-quite-right partners?

The most common reason for seeking other partners—not to be confused with the most common excuse, "I need some space"—is a desire for new flesh, a new body to make love with. Even though people's bodies change—not always for the better—as they get older, chances are you found yourself on the slippery trail headed toward sexual oblivion long before you rolled over in bed and discovered a shriveled up old body lying next to you.

If you're like most men, the real reason for "straying" was not because the "body at home" was starting to fall apart, but rather because your *attitude* about "the body at home" was falling apart. The first mistake was to try to have a relationship with someone whom you looked at only as a body.

Attitude and concentration play a big part in this whole cycle of events. When you meet someone new, you are willing, for whatever rea-

son, to concentrate totally on that person. You devote time and energy to creating a relationship with that person, whether it's making sure that you talk with her, going out of your way to arrange something that you think she might find enjoyable, or buying her a gift. All the while, your attitude is extremely receptive toward this other person, overlooking faults and withholding criticism.

Now what would happen if you did this with that "body at home"? You say, "Well, she doesn't do this" or "She doesn't do that." What about *you?* One of the key reasons you're probably so hot for the "next in line" is because of what *you're* doing. *You* are the one who is providing the heat to fuel that passion. *You* are interested. *You* are concentrating on the positive aspects of that other person and not being critical. *You* are the one who is creating something between you and someone else.

We have a peculiar attitude regarding relationships. We have a tendency to assume that because sex is a natural function, relationships are natural also. And if they occur naturally, then once they've formed, we don't have to do

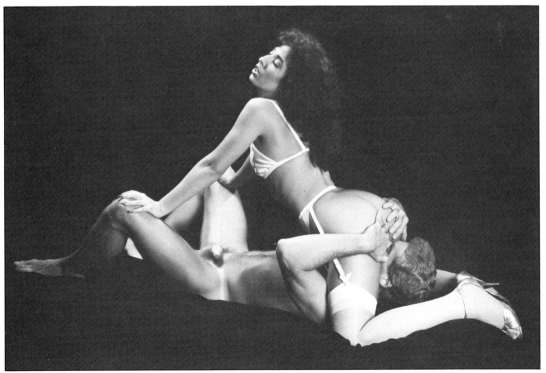

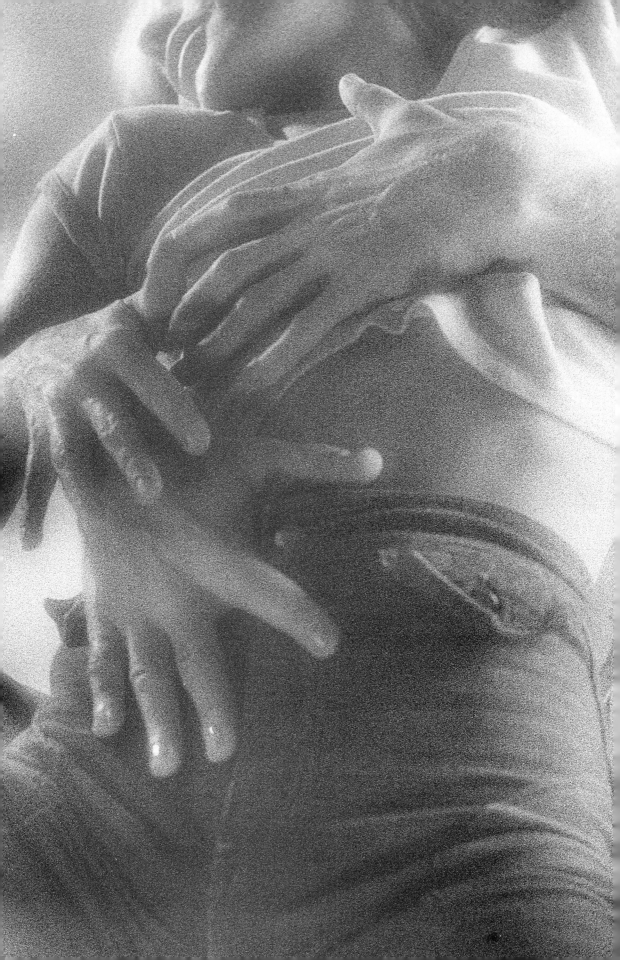

anything about them. We just put them on autopilot. As a woman once said to me, during one of our too-frequent disagreements, "If we have to work so hard at our relationship, that must mean that the relationship isn't worth saving."

The truth is that every relationship needs working at now and then if it's going to survive. It is not written in stone that once a relationship starts out on the right foot, all responsibility for it should be abandoned. Anyone who has had an extended relationship recognizes the importance—the necessity—of working at it. This work is not without its rewards. Indeed, there is a special kind of satisfaction in working out problems that other people cannot seem to handle. Coming out the other end can often profoundly deepen mutual appreciation and respect—and these, more than anything anyone can do with a sex organ, are what successful relationships are built upon.

Why discuss attitude in a book about love-making? One reason is perspective. You can use this book in much the same way as one uses a booklet of instructions on how to put together a swing set. That is your prerogative. Or you may use it to improve not only your sexual technique, but your ability to relate to the person, or persons, with whom you make love.

Another reason is that attitude, while not the whole ball game, may well be a good six or seven innings of it. Consider this incident related to me recently by a 26-year-old friend of mine.

"It was the most amazing thing. As you know, I've been thinking of leaving Jenny, and mainly because our sex just hasn't been, you know, up to par. In fact, it's been downright boring. So, I've been looking around and I've had an eye on this secretary at work.

"Anyhow, Jenny and I went down to La Jolla last weekend to see her folks. She and I went to a little bar downtown to have a few drinks. To be honest, I was as bored as usual and watching every young thing in sight—and there were plenty that had me salivating.

"About 11:30 we left the bar and walked a couple of blocks to a parking garage where I'd parked the car. As we were walking down a flight of stairs, I happened to bump into Jenny because she was having trouble opening the

door and I wasn't paying attention. As I bumped into her, my hand pressed against her dress, which was made of a light summer material, and I felt that she wasn't wearing anything except string-bikini underwear underneath. I started rubbing her ass and I gradually reached up under her dress to feel her pussy—which was so wet that her underwear was almost soaked. She started to moan and become beautifully responsive. I lifted her dress and, as I did, I realized that at any moment someone might come through the door we were standing against or the door that was one flight above. But I didn't have time to think about it too much because Jenny was already unzipping my pants.

"I looked down at Jenny's body—her tanned legs shaped nicely by her high-heeled shoes, her small but firm breasts, her luscious lips—and I was knocked out by her. When I got inside her, it was incredible—for her and for me. We made love there for about five minutes and then went home and had one of the longest and best lovemaking sessions we've ever had.

"The next morning, Jenny fixed me breakfast in bed—after which we made love again. That afternoon we went to the beach and I took some pictures. I got them developed the next day and took one to work and put it on my desk. I even called several of my friends' attention to the picture of 'my girlfriend.' I was so proud of her, and I felt more for her than I'd felt in years. And to think that just a couple of days before I was bored with her. I'm glad I wised up before I lost her."

What does this story tell you? Had Jenny changed? Had she become more beautiful? No. Only one thing had changed: her boyfriend's attitude. One day he was bored with her and didn't look at her as sexually attractive. The next day he looked at her and saw a beautiful, sexy woman whom he was so proud of that he wanted to show her picture off to his friends.

My friend in the previous story was lucky. Most of us don't appreciate what we've got till it's gone. When that person you didn't think you loved isn't around when you turn out the lights, that's often the first time you give it any thought.

How many times have your relationships or potentially satisfying evenings fallen victim to a

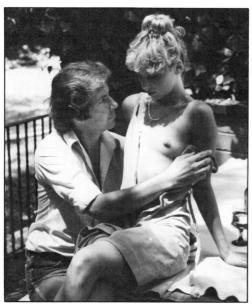

lackadaisical attitude? Marcus Aurelius said, "Our lives are what our thoughts make them." So are our relationships.

MOOD AND SETTING

Sex without mood and setting can be likened to players with bats, balls, and gloves who don't have a field on which to play. Most of us think more of mood and setting when we're dating. That's the time for candlelight dinners and dimly lit bedrooms with appropriate music. After the dating period, most people don't think about mood and setting except for special occasions such as birthdays and anniversaries.

Well, if it works for those occasions, why not give it a try sometime out of the blue when you just want to inject a little something different into the sexual mix? That's exactly what Robert S. did.

"My wife and I both work, and we're usually pretty tired by the time we get home, which is about seven o'clock, so we often just meet at home and go out to a restaurant for dinner. We live in Westwood, which is about ten minutes from the Pacific Ocean. For years we'd talked about having an intimate dinner on the beach, but we never did it.

"I decided that our relationship could use a little livening up, so I planned an oceanside dinner and didn't tell her anything about it,

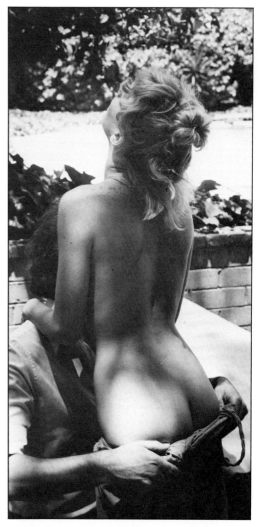

except that I was planning to take her out to dinner. I bought her favorite wine, chilled it, and put it in ice in the trunk of the car minutes before we left. I filled a small picnic basket with grapes, three different kinds of cheese, olives, fresh-sliced bread, a checkered table cloth, a corkscrew, napkins, plates, utensils, two candlesticks, candles, and matches.

"She still had no idea what was going on, even while we were driving to the beach—she thought we were just going to a restaurant near the beach. When I drove into the beach parking lot, she looked at me with a very confused look. Then, when I had her get out of the car and I opened up the trunk and showed her the

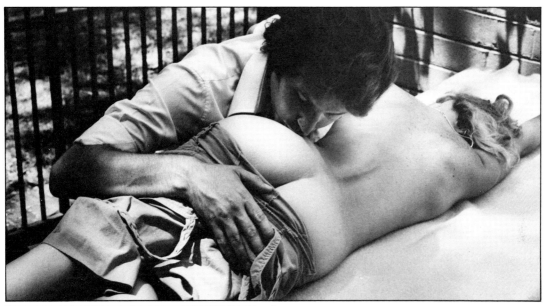

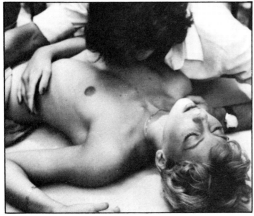

picnic basket, with a card I'd picked up for her taped to the lid, her face lit up like a kid's on Christmas morning.

"We spread the tablecloth and picnicked about fifty feet from the ocean as the sun went down. Seeing Linda in that setting—her hair blown free about her shoulders by the sea breeze, her face profiled against the setting sun—awakened in me feelings for her that I'd forgotten about. One of the really interesting things about the whole experience was that I thought I was doing something that would make Linda happy, that she would enjoy. And though she really did enjoy it, I enjoyed doing at least as much as she enjoyed

having it done for her.

"Our dinner on the ocean ended perfectly when I planted the candlesticks in the sand and lit the candles. I retrieved two sweaters from the car and we finished off the bottle of wine, lying in each other's arms, lit by candlelight, the smell and the sound of the ocean filling our senses.

"After about an hour, I blew out the candles and, wrapping ourselves in the tablecloth, we made love to each other for another hour. Then we adjourned to the privacy of our bedroom."

Maybe you don't live near the Pacific Ocean, and maybe you don't like picnics and wine. But surely if you put your mind to it, if you really wanted to, you could create a scenario that would provide the stimulus for a romantic evening with your partner. So often we wait for others, or for events and circumstances outside ourselves, to take control of our lives or to change them for the better.

If you're waiting for your partner to become more sexy, or to do something, or to change in some way that will make you feel better about your relationship, chances are you're going to be waiting a long time. Usually, there's just one person who can make you feel better about your relationship, and that's you. And you might just find that playing with the mood and setting of your relationship a little now and then will cut down your waiting time considerably.

FEMALE · ANATOMY

That we don't really know much about female anatomy, or sexual anatomy and function in general, is just another example of the sexual ignorance of our culture. Most men know more about their cars and their computers than they do about their wives' vulva. Ask most men what a vulva is, and they'll tell you it's a well-built Swedish car.

To make matters worse, most women don't know a whole lot more about the function of—sometimes even the look of—their sex organs. There are many reasons for this, most of them cultural—the result of male-dominated societies creating "taboos" that all but legislated against women gaining control of their own sexuality.

In many cases women believed, and some still believe today, that their vulvas are ugly. Although that may sound preposterous in a supposedly enlightened sexual age, sex researchers from Freud right on through to contemporary therapists confirm that many women still harbor concerns about the appearance of their sex organs. This real-life story from Sue H. illustrates how such anxieties can affect a relationship.

"Though John was not my first lover, he was the first man with whom I'd had a warm and loving relationship. He would always want to communicate when we had a problem, and it didn't take me long to realize what a difference communicating—really communicating, not just talking—can make.

"He noticed that whenever we made love, I always wanted the lights off. Also, I would never allow him to give me head. I was always willing to walk around the house with just my bikini bottoms on, but never completely nude.

"After about a month, John sat me down and asked me why I never wanted him to see my vagina. At first I denied that I was trying to hide my vagina, but he prodded me to tell the truth. By then I knew that John was someone I could talk to about my hang-ups. I told him that I thought my vagina was ugly and that I was embarrassed for him to see it. I could see that John stifled a laugh because he knew I was serious. He told me that he understood.

"That night John lit candles in the bedroom, so it wasn't really bright, but our bodies were clearly lit by the candlelight. After a minimal amount of resistance from me, John took my

panties down and moved his head down between my legs. He gently parted my legs and started softly caressing my labia and clitoris. He said things like 'Sue, you're so pretty between your legs, I can't imagine why you would want to cover it up.' And, 'You have the most beautiful pussy I've ever seen.'

"By this time, I was so wet that I lost all inhibition. When his tongue touched my clit, I just about exploded with one of the best orgasms I've ever had in my life.

"Since then, I've actually become proud of how my vagina looks and the wonderful effect its appearance has on John. He has even started 'taking care' of my vagina by trimming the hair occasionally and brushing it with a tiny hairbrush he bought just for that purpose."

Sue had bought into a ridiculous myth that her vagina was ugly. It was totally untrue. All it took was somebody to tell her it was beautiful.

The female sexual anatomy (See page 17) is composed of the labia majora, labia minora, vagina, and clitoris. These components together are often referred to as the vulva (also known as the pussy or vagina depending on one's preference).

The mysteries surrounding the vulva—its secret powers, its beauty—serve as powerful magnets, pulling men to it. But although mystery is good for erotic effect, a little can go a long way. As previously discussed, research into sexual matters has never been high on the list of priorities of modern culture. Therefore, myth and mystery far outweigh fact and substance.

Here are a few facts.

The labia are the inner and outer lips of the vulva. The outer lips are called the labia majora, the inner lips the labia minora. The labia majora are generally covered with hair and serve as covering or protection for the labia minora and the clitoris, as well as the opening into the vagina.

The labia minora are folds of skin, or lips, that contain a network of nerves and are therefore extremely sensitive to stimulation. At their uppermost point they form a "hood" that partially covers the clitoris. In some women these inner lips are visible, while in other women they remain covered by the labia majora until stimulation reveals them. Either situation is completely normal. Because the labia minora are so sensi-

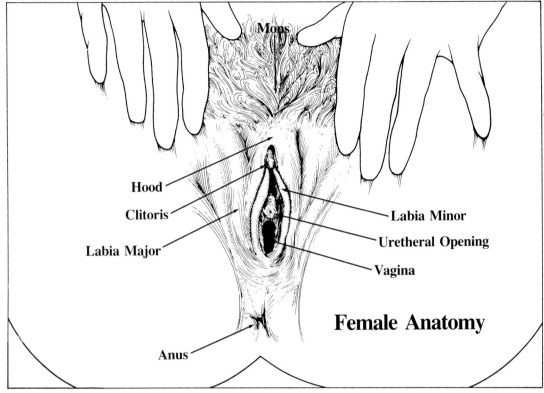

Mons

Hood

Clitoris

Labia Major

Labia Minor

Uretheral Opening

Vagina

Female Anatomy

Anus

tive to stimulation, they should be targeted by the man during lovemaking, particularly during foreplay.

The clitoris is located just above the exit of the urethra, near the vaginal opening, where the labia minora join together at their uppermost point. It is small and highly sensitive. It can usually be seen between the folds of the outer labia. As with the penis, the clitoris is made of erectile tissue that is highly sensitive to stimulation. It reacts strongly and immediately to touch and becomes larger and harder the more sexually excited the woman becomes.

If there is a sexual nerve center, this is it. A lover who wishes to please his female partner will find it necessary to become familiar with his lover's clitoris. As with the penis, not every clitoris is alike. They differ in size and sensitivity.

One fact that is not commonly known is that the clitoris actually recedes under the hood shortly before orgasm, just as the woman is building to climax. If clitoral stimulation is not maintained, the woman can be left "hanging on the edge" of an orgasm. A woman with a longer

clitoris will still have enough of it exposed, even after the clitoris withdraws, so that stimulation is not interrupted. But a woman with a shorter clitoris may need to communicate this phenomenon to her lover. A man who observes symptoms of this phenomenon—his female partner becoming aroused, building to a climax, then not being able to make it "over the top"—should investigate to find out if a short clitoris might be the problem. If so, the solution is really quite simple. Maintain stimulation of the clitoris, even if through the hood, whether manually, orally, or with a position that allows for uninterrupted stimulation.

The vagina is a narrow, elastic canal, surrounded by muscular tissues, leading from the external genital orifice to the uterus. It is approximately eight to ten centimeters long and is always coated with secretion. This secretion increases greatly during arousal, thus allowing the penis to penetrate more easily. The vagina's primary function during intercourse is to allow penile penetration and to conduct the subsequent ejaculation toward the ovaries.

The walls of the vagina are muscular, and the elasticity of the vagina varies from woman to woman. It has generally been assumed that young girls have "tighter" vaginas and that after considerable sexual activity, and particularly after childbirth, the vagina "loosens up," never to return to its "tightened" state.

However, recent scientific evidence has cast this idea more in the role of myth than fact. In Great Britain a study was conducted involving young women who were virgins, women who had sex regularly, women who had given birth, and older women who had never had sexual intercourse. A balloon device was inserted into the vagina while the participants squeezed their PC muscles (see chapter on PC MUSCLE) as hard as they could.

The study's findings often ran counter to contemporary thinking on the subject of PC-muscle strength. Many of the women who had given birth were able to exert more pressure on the balloon than the older women who had never had intercourse. Many of the women who had given birth (& not done PC-muscle exercises) were able to exert more pressure than their counterparts who had done PC-muscle exercises after giving birth.

Why? The only common denominator among the women who were "tighter" was exercise—not specific exercises designed to strengthen the PC muscle, but exercise in general. Doctors involved in the study suggested that exercise, particularly aerobics and other exercises currently in vogue at local workout clubs, serves to indirectly work and strengthen the muscles in the lower abdominal area.

If the findings of this preliminary study prove out, not only will the current exercise trend make us healthier, it may prove to be a boon for increased sexual pleasure as well. For now, our advice to a woman who wishes to retain vaginal "tightness" would be to perform a regimen that includes *both* regular abdominal exercises *and* traditional PC-muscle-strengthening exercises.

GROOMING THE PUBIC HAIR

While a woman may spend an hour in the bathroom fixing her hair for a date, she can go an entire lifetime without considering the possibility of enhancing the look of her vulva by experimenting with different "pubic hairstyles." Just as a different hairstyle will accentuate or play down different aspects of the face, so too will different pubic hairstyles accentuate or cover certain aspects of the vulva.

Today's woman, who spends a lot of time in high-cut bathing suits and leotards, is more aware than ever of the necessity of shaving or shaping pubic hair. Some women shave their pubic hair from the clitoris down, not only to allow their lovers easy access to the clitoris, but also because their lovers may be more turned on by the sight of the labia and clitoris than by a clump of hair that obscures them.

It is not uncommon these days for women to shave their pubic hair entirely. Although this could be a turn-off for some men, many men are extremely aroused by the sight of a totally unadorned vulva. Shaving the pubic area requires regular daily or every other day shaving in order to keep it smooth; otherwise the resulting "stubble" can make intercourse quite uncomfortable.

Some women prefer to take a less drastic course of action, choosing to shave their pubic hair in the shape of a heart or in some other way scale down the amount of hair. Regardless of the approach, shaving the pubic hair is not an irreversible act. If you or your lover doesn't like it, the hair will always grow back.

There are basically three ways of removing pubic hair. Shaving with a razor is the most common method. If you're shaving for the first time, you'll need a pair of scissors to cut away the bulk of the hair before you can use shaving cream and a razor. Be sure to use a new, sharp razor.

The second method is to use a hair-removal cream. As with the first method, this requires regular use because the hair always grows back. Also, you may want to check with your doctor before using a chemical product on so sensitive an area as your vulva.

The third method is by plucking or electrolysis. Plucking can be extremely time-consuming and slightly painful but, once accomplished, lasts much longer than the first two methods. Electrolysis can be expensive, but the results are permanent. Of course, you need to be certain that you want a clean-shaven pubic area before going forward with electrolysis.

MALE·ANATOMY

Another vast realm of mystery, myth, and misinformation is, of course, the male sex organ. Entire cultures have been built around the phallus, and there are some who would argue that contemporary society, albeit not as blatant as some previous societies, is not so far removed from our phallus-worshipping ancestors.

Is there a man alive who has not experienced, at one time or another, some anxiety about his penis—its size, shape, circumference, or what have you? Even though contemporary literature insists that "it's the magician, not the wand" that counts, penis anxieties still abound. Witness the story of Paul T.

"I'd just broken up with my girlfriend, and I was starting to date. My girlfriend and I had been going together for about five years, from the time we were both 18, so almost all of my sexual experience had been with her.

"I knew that she was dating other guys after we split up, and for the first time the thought occurred to me: how do I measure up? The thought of my old girlfriend making love with other men and comparing me to them increased my anxiety. By the time I started dating again, I was almost to the point where I would try to avoid situations that might lead to intercourse. I would become anxious and embarrassed if a woman even touched me for fear that she might reach between my legs and feel a penis that,

when unaroused, was quite small. For a while, I stopped dating altogether.

"John, my oldest and best friend, and I had known each other since junior high and had roomed together in college. At the time of my separation from my girlfriend, we belonged to the same health club. Being roommates and having showered together many times at the gym and in school locker rooms, I'd had numerous opportunities to observe the size of John's penis, which, to my eye, was quite large. During this particular period in my life, I actually became envious of the size of John's penis.

"When I turned down a date with a girl I'd been wanting to go out with for some time, I realized that something had to be done. I didn't know any sex therapists, and I wasn't certain if anything that drastic was required. All I knew was that I had to do something.

"So I decided to talk about my anxieties with my friend John. Our friendship had weathered lots of rough times, we'd shared each other's innermost secrets, and we had never betrayed that trust. One night after working out, we went out to have a few drinks, and I told him what was on my mind. To my surprise, he told me that my worries were common and that he too had had similar concerns. In fact, he told me that after reading an article in *Playboy* about penis size, he actually took out a tape measure

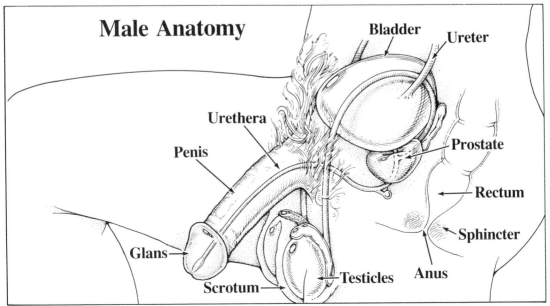

Male Anatomy

Bladder
Ureter
Urethera
Penis
Prostate
Rectum
Sphincter
Glans
Scrotum
Testicles
Anus

and measured his erect penis. The tape read six-and-a-quarter inches, which according to the article was toward the high end of the normal range—five-and-a-half to six-and-a-half inches. He told me that different positions compensated for most size differences between men's and women's sex organs, and he went on to tell me about several. Finally he closed with the familiar "it's not what you've got but how you use it" routine. To be honest, that was just about what I'd expected him to say, so it didn't really make me feel any better.

"When I returned home that night, it occurred to me to measure my own erect penis. Initially, I was afraid to do so because I knew I was going to 'weigh in' as a flyweight, and since such a measurement would be an objective test, I could no longer allow myself the luxury of believing my penis to be of average length.

"However, a couple of nights later my curiosity got the better of me, and I took out a tape measure my old girlfriend had left behind, stimulated myself to an erection, and measured my penis. Guess what? It was just a little over six inches.

"I was ecstatic to know that I was average—whatever that really means. Shortly afterward, I spoke to a friend of mine who was in med school, and he told me that one of the most debilitating misconceptions about penis size is one that is fostered in locker rooms. That is, most guys believe that if the guy next to you has a schlong that hangs down about four or five inches, he's automatically going to have a much larger erection than the guy whose penis is only a couple or three inches long when limp. The truth is, erection proves to be the great equalizer. Don't get me wrong, I'm not saying that all penises are the same length. But according to my doctor friend, most of the penises that appear to be much shorter when flaccid compare favorably with their long-when-limp counterparts when both are fully erect.

"Since that time, I haven't worried about the size of my penis. Rather, I've concentrated on being sensitive to my partner's desires and on my own technique for satisfying those desires."

Lack of experience is the most common reason for such anxieties—that plus a variety of myths and jokes such as, "Hey, that looks like a penis, only smaller." Although it is true that penises vary in size, color, and shape, it is most definitely also true that experience in all aspects of lovemaking skills can compensate for virtually anything a man may lack in penis size.

The most noticeable difference in the way a penis looks is whether or not it is circumcised. Circumcision involves the removal of the foreskin from the penis. This procedure usually takes place shortly after birth, though it can be done later in life, and may be performed for religious reasons or hygienic ones—that is, because it prevents the accumulation of unwanted substances often found under the foreskin in uncircumcised males. Although it has been suspected that circumcision decreases sensitivity, this is generally untrue.

The length and circumference of the penis vary from man to man. The size of an erect penis cannot be determined from its limp state, as was illustrated in Paul's story. During arousal, cavities in the penis shaft fill with blood, thus hardening, or stiffening, the penis. This process is an involuntary physical manifestation of erotic thought or physical stimulation.

At the top of the penis is the glans, commonly referred to as the "head." It is the most sensitive part of the male sex organ and, when stimulated, brings an orgasm.

One irony that has been lost on most of the male population, though well known to sex researchers for years, is that of the possible groups—men with unusually large penises, men with average-size penises, and men with small penises—men with large penises have the most difficult time finding acceptable partners. Women can stretch or contract to accommodate the average man and even the smaller man. The smaller man can use various manual and oral methods plus certain positions to satisfy his mate and can satisfy himself completely between the legs of his lover. However, the unusually large man may not be able to satisfy himself between his lover's legs unless he finds a woman who has an unusually large vagina. For the man with a large penis, only this type of woman can afford him the vehicle needed for optimum sexual release.

Research indicates that a woman enjoys looking at and caressing her lover's penis. Therefore, it is a good idea to take care of the way your penis looks, smells, and feels. There are many good hygienic reasons for doing this as well. If a man expects his partner's sex organs to be clean and to smell good, he should give his lover the same consideration. Whereas a heavy musky smell can often do wonders for sexual excitement, if that musky fragrance weighs too heavily, bordering on or becoming the pungent odor of uncleanliness, it can have a negative effect on lovemaking. Listen to the story of Toni B.

"My boyfriend, Eddy, and I had been going together for about three or four months and I still had not given him head. Don't get me wrong, I really wanted to. He's got a beautiful cock and I used to fantasize about going down on him and taking the whole thing down my throat—I knew I could do that because I used to 'deep-throat' my ex-boyfriend all the time. The problem was, Eddy never showered before we had sex.

"I know this sounds like a minor thing and that I should have said something right away. But sometimes you think you might be hurting somebody's feelings. If you think I'm wrong, just consider how difficult it is to tell somebody he's got bad breath, and then you'll have some idea of how hard it might be to tell someone his cock smells bad.

"Eddy wore tight pants and he sweated a lot, so there was a reason why he always had a heavy odor in his crotch, but the whole thing could have been taken care of if he just washed before we had sex.

"Finally, one afternoon after we'd come back from the beach, I pulled Eddy into the shower with me. After washing his cock very thoroughly myself, I gave him an afternoon to remember.

"When we were through, he told me how much he enjoyed my giving him head and he asked me why I'd never done it before. I finally broke down and told him. And you know, he took it great. He told me that I should have just told him in the first place and that he would have understood. Now showering is part of Eddy's routine before coming to bed. I'm happy that he does it. And he's even happier about it than I am."

So often couples are just a few hard-to-speak words away from achieving the kind of compatibility they desire in a relationship.

It should be added here that even the man with the best "equipment" can occasionally suffer "equipment failure." In a society as stress-laden as the one we live in, stress can, and often does, affect our attitude, our physical health, and sometimes our sexual performance.

Regardless of all the barroom talk to the contrary, there is hardly a man alive who hasn't experienced failure to attain an erection. It can be a confidence-shattering experience. What that man needs to do is get right back "in the saddle" and ride. Paradoxically, that is the one thing that may frighten him the most.

It is important for the female partner to understand the situation, to avoid blowing it out of proportion, and to be comforting rather than demanding. Stress is something we need to learn to cope with, and when it affects life in the bedroom, we must learn to cope with that, too.

Among the ways of dealing with this problem is to enter the female while limp. Many men are not aware of certain positions that, as long as the female is well lubricated, allow the man to insert his penis even though it is not erect. For example, the woman lies on her back and hooks her hands under and around her knees. She spreads her legs and pulls them back, sometimes even to the point of lifting her lower back off the bed slightly. This position exposes the vulva completely to the man. When he approaches her from between her legs, he is able to insert even a limp penis into the well-lubricated labia and vagina. Once inside, the "importance" and "necessity" of achieving an erection are lessened and the anxiety level decreases.

This method undercuts the anxiety of trying to achieve an erection in order to prove one's masculinity. Most men know the torment of going through all the motions of foreplay with a lover, concentrating only on whether or not they can achieve an erection. Such fixation is counterproductive in every possible way. First, the man is concentrating on himself and not his lover. Second, he's turning his attention away from the very stimuli that usually cause him to have an erection. Is it any wonder that an erection rarely occurs under such circumstances?

As a man gets older, stress and age take their toll. But as long as he has a partner who is understanding and loving, any problems arising from these causes are small indeed.

THE · PC · MUSCLE

Whereas men tend to have anxieties about their penises being too small, women tend to be concerned that their vaginas are too big. Typical jokes revolve around losing large objects, such as trucks, in the vagina. The only thing that really gets lost is a woman's confidence in her ability to satisfy her lover. Listen to the story of Helen Y.

"Sex with my husband, Bobby, took a drastic turn for the worse immediately after our first child was born. There's no doubt that a certain amount of stretching had taken place, and we could both 'feel the difference' between what our sex used to be like and what it was like after I gave birth.

"My mother told me that the same thing had happened to her and that Bobby and I would simply have to resign ourselves to the new circumstances. 'Besides,' she said, 'you have a new baby to keep you busy.' My mother had never been one for sage advice regarding sex. Anyway, it wasn't me I was worried about—although I missed sex the way it used to be, too—I was worried about Bobby. After all, he was a normal, healthy, good-looking guy. He was nice about the change in our sexual relations, but I felt very insecure about it and became obsessed with the idea that it would just be a matter of time until he found someone else.

"I spoke with my girlfriend, Julie, about my 'problem,' and she said that she had gone through a similar problem after her first child. She told me that her gynecologist had given her exercises to do that would strengthen her PC muscle. She said that in no time she regained most, if not all, of her prechildbirth form. She described the exercises to me, and I started doing them several times every day.

"A few weeks later, after we'd made love one night, Bobby made the comment that he thought my vagina was contracting back to its original size. That was all the encouragement I needed. I've been doing the exercises ever since—about three years. Bobby is happy with what he calls his 'tight pussy,' and I'm enjoying sex as much as or more than I ever have."

So where and what is this PC (pubococcygeal) muscle? Both men and women have a PC muscle. It is located in the pelvic region, about an inch under the skin, and is shaped like a figure 8. A simple way to identify the PC muscle is to picture yourself urinating and hearing the phone ring before you are finished. The muscle you use to stop urinating is the PC muscle.

The more toned this muscle is, the more control the woman has in "grasping" the man's penis. Naturally, this significantly increases the man's pleasure, both because the vagina feels tighter, and also because of the additional sensation of having his penis rhythmically or erratically squeezed by the vagina.

PC MUSCLE EXERCISES FOR WOMEN

Like any other muscle in the body, the PC muscle responds to exercise and becomes lax and out of shape with nonuse.

After locating the PC muscle, tighten it, then release it. Make sure you don't use any other muscles while you're squeezing the PC muscle. Isolate it, then use it. Moving your legs apart slightly will help you isolate the PC muscle.

Start your exercise program by performing this exercise six times a day for a week. Tighten the PC muscle for a few seconds, then release it. Do this ten times at each session. The great thing about this exercise is that you don't have to buy any special workout clothes or join a gym. You might say that the gym is between your legs. You can perform this exercise while sitting in traffic, watching TV with your family, or sitting at your desk at work. Nobody knows what you're doing—for some this will be an added erotic bonus.

The second week, make some changes in your routine. First, instead of ten exercises at a session, make it twenty. Second, instead of tensing, holding, then releasing, this time tense and release quickly ten times, thus creating a "fluttering" sensation. Don't be surprised if your stamina for such an exercise is not considerable in the beginning. However, you'll be rewarded by continuing to perform this exercise diligently because the PC muscle, like any other muscle, will respond to continued exercise. By the time you get to fifty contractions and flutters per session, you'll be ready to take your lover to heaven and back.

As in the development of any muscle that was once underdeveloped, you will find that you can do things with your developed PC muscle that you were not able to do previously. For example, you can now squeeze your lover's

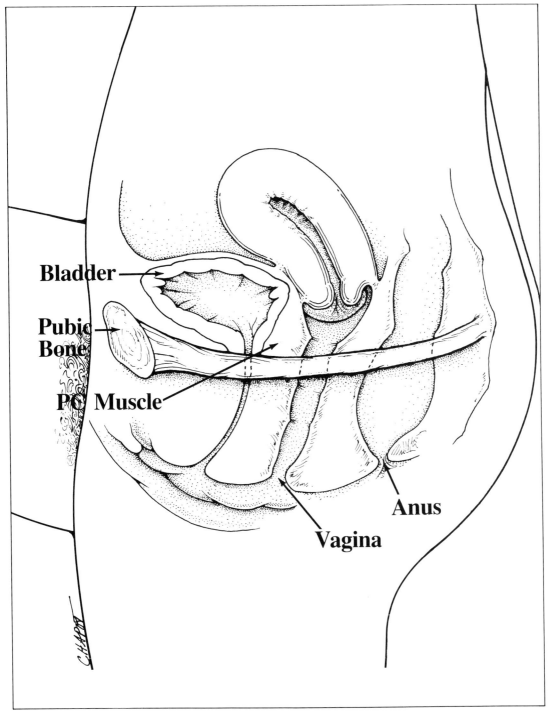

Bladder

Pubic Bone

PC Muscle

Vagina

Anus

Female PC Muscle

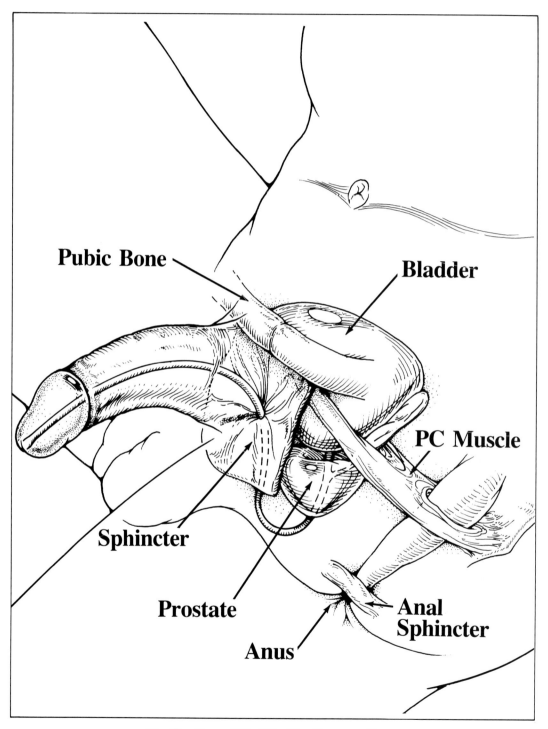

Pubic Bone

Bladder

PC Muscle

Sphincter

Prostate

Anal Sphincter

Anus

Male PC Muscle

penis on the in-stroke, which makes it more difficult for him to enter you—a difficulty he will undoubtedly not complain about too loudly. This action will have the effect of stretching the penile skin back from the top, which will considerably heighten his sensation. You can squeeze on the out-stroke, which will keep him inside you for a little longer, and then tighten just a little extra as the head gets close to the vaginal opening. This will put pressure on that sensitive area right at the edge of the vagina. Try squeezing to different rhythms—your favorite lovemaking song, your heartbeat, the pulse of your lover's throbbing cock.

Lying still with your lover's penis inside you might be the ideal time to squeeze a little, then a little more, and a little more, rhythmically, until you drive your man wild. Instruct him to lie perfectly still until you tell him to move. He may not want to do so immediately, but after he feels what you have in store for him, he'll gladly accede to your wishes.

If physical exercise is not your thing, small electronic machines, which look somewhat like dildos, are available that will electronically stimulate the PC muscle for you.

PC MUSCLE EXERCISES FOR MEN

First, locate and isolate the PC muscle (remember, it's the muscle you use to stop urinating when the phone rings). For your exercises, you will need to be alone, and you will need a handkerchief or light towel. Now, caress yourself until you have reached a strong erection. Stand up and drape the cloth over your erect penis. Contract the PC muscle rhythmically so that the towel moves up and down. If you happen to live with your parents and decide to perform this exercise, it is wise to do it in a room with a door you can lock. This is a most difficult exercise to explain to a casual observer. As you become more accustomed to the feel of contracting your PC muscle, you can do away with the towel and simply perform the exercise *au naturel*.

Once you have strengthened the PC muscle, try it out with your lover. Pause while you are deep inside her, then start squeezing your PC muscle. Your penis will stiffen and swell, and she'll love the feeling this causes inside her vagina. It will create a sensual contrast to the usual in-out thrusting.

If you're lucky enough to have a lover who has also strengthened her PC muscle, you will be able to give each other pleasure that you never knew existed. Lie still in a position that keeps some leverage or pressure on the penis, then start contracting your PC muscle. Do not speak or move anything else but the PC muscle. Allow your lover to respond by squeezing her PC muscle. "Speak" to each other in the language of love, massaging each other with your sex organs. It's a thrill you won't likely forget, and it can make an excellent addition to your lovemaking repertoire. Just ask Robert H.

"My girlfriend read about how to perform PC-muscle exercises in one of her women's magazines. The article also said that men could do basically the same exercise in order to develop muscle control over their penises. We work out a lot together—we jog every morning for about thirty minutes, and we both belong to the same gym where we take about three classes a week together. So we decided to both learn the PC muscle exercises and see what happened.

"Soon we both noticed that we were developing more strength and control—she over her vaginal muscles, and I over the muscles that control the movement of my penis. Gradually we started to incorporate this muscle control into our regular sexual activity.

"One night while we were making love, I got into a sitting position, legs crossed Indian-style in front of me. I moved my girlfriend into a position so that she was on my lap, facing me, legs locked around my waist. I positioned her body slightly so that enough downward pressure was still being exerted on my penis so that I would retain a taut erection.

"Then we both started to squeeze our PC muscles. We'd been doing the exercises for about a month, and we'd already noticed a gradual strengthening. I squeezed, then she squeezed. I squeezed twice, then she squeezed twice. We started to develop a rhythm, back and forth. It was incredible. In fact, we both were able to come at the same time, without any thrusting movements. All the while I was looking in her eyes, just squeezing my PC muscle. It was a wonderful way to have an orgasm— almost peaceful, serene, but very, very sexy."

DRESSING AND UNDRESSING FOR SEX

When I was about 8 years old, three of my friends and I set out on a quest that was to take us into the uncharted—for us—waters of female anatomy. Our goal was to find out what a naked woman looked like. To understand the challenge of this, you must put yourself in a time machine and transport yourself back to a time when female nudity was not readily visible on television, at the beach, or at supermarket checkout stands. *Playboy* was not yet acceptable coffee table literature. In short, it was the dark ages.

The only magazine my friends and I could find at the time that pertained even vaguely to our pursuit was *National Geographic*. A bizarre side effect of this research tool was the conclusion that white women had no breasts.

Censorship in the 1950s and early '60s seemed omnipresent. How many times we got so close to seeing naked women, only to find those nasty black marks over the target areas! It was a sweet agony because we knew that just below those black marks were the very treasures of our quest.

As we geared up our efforts to find out exactly what a naked woman looked like, we encountered an even more formidable obstacle—the airbrush. One member of our group brought in a photograph that purported to

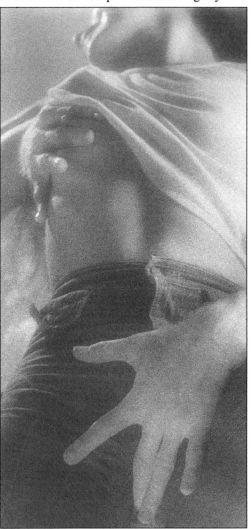

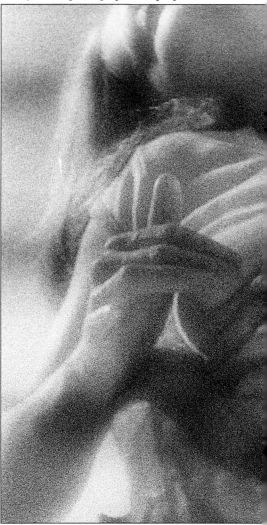

capture a full frontal view of a naked woman. Though the breasts were visible—thank god—the woman in the photograph was totally smooth "down there." At first, such photographs led to a myriad of rather major, and potentially dangerous, misconceptions regarding the actual makeup of the female anatomy.

Finally, after nearly a year of frustration and betrayal—by censors and airbrushers—one group member brought in a real photograph of a naked lady. It was a time for rejoicing and mutual congratulations.

Our real initiation, however, came some years later as it had for several generations of men before us—at the local burlesque house. Seeing

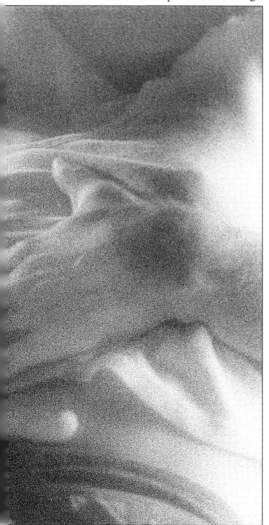

a black-and-white photograph was one thing, but seeing a real naked lady—well, that was something entirely different.

Our entire gang sneaked into the Town Hall Burlesque Theater to see Alexandra the Great. Now there was a woman! As I think back on the experience, I have the distinct feeling that the ticket taker wasn't fooled when all of us—who just happened to be at various stages of 16 at the time—told him we were 18. So as not to be too obvious, naturally we all sat in the first row.

I can still recall my excitement and arousal as Alexandra took off her gloves, unzipped her dress, and stood there in high heels, stockings,

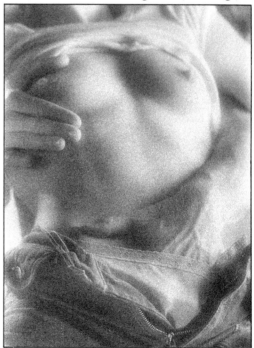

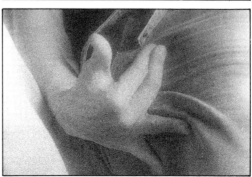

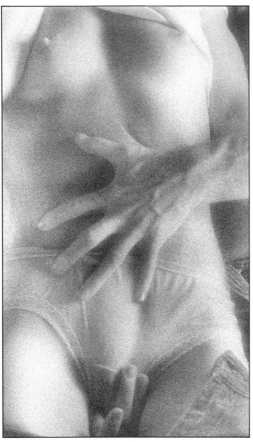

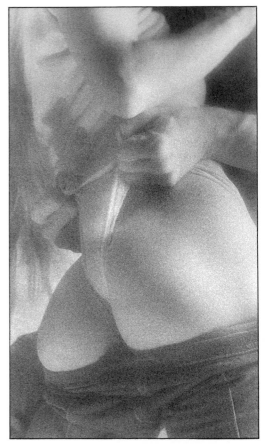

garter belt, and boa, her erect nipples sticking straight out and bouncing slightly with every sultry movement. If I had to compare her body to the sexy bodies I've seen since then, I'd have to say that it was only adequate. But the way she revealed that body, highlighted it, and "offered" it to us made her look like the sexiest woman in the world. All things considered, she'd have to rank right up there even now.

If you believe that the clothing you wear and how you remove that clothing makes no difference in the lovemaking art, you need look no further than the time-honored tradition of strippers. In order to give a sense of balance to this idea, consider the "male exotic dancer" craze. Have you ever seen the reaction of the women at these shows? They're animals, really—more so than any burlesque-show audience I've ever seen.

The point is, a woman likes to see her man dress sexily, and she enjoys either watching him

undress or the pleasure of undressing him herself.

Women know how aroused they can get by seeing a man in a nicely tailored suit or a tight pair of jeans. Most men have had the experience of being knocked out by the turn of a calf in a pair of stockings, or swept away at the beach by the way a bathing suit reveals a tight pair of buns. And we've all had the experience of not being as thrilled as we thought we'd be when those "trappings" were finally stripped away. In short, the sexily adorned body is often much more titillating than the totally nude body.

Smart dressers know how to dress. They are honest about their strong points and their weaknesses, and they dress to highlight their strengths and downplay their weaknesses.

Chances are, the first time you made love with your girlfriend or wife you had to struggle with a zipper or two. And even though you did, everything probably turned out all right. Now you most likely just meet in bed, totally nude, and make love. Sometime soon, just for a change of pace, try a little foreplay with your clothes on. It'll probably bring back pleasant memories, and you just may find it extremely erotic.

Many men have fond and erotic memories of sitting in a dark movie theater with a date, an arm around her shoulder, a finger inching its way toward a breast—pure exhilaration. And what man cannot recall some wonderful incidents of slipping a hand under a dress and up a smooth thigh toward . . .

All these experiences involve—in fact, require—clothing. Clothing has taken an undeserved bad rap as far as sexuality goes.

Hardly any thinking person can pass up a good mystery. You're given the facts and the puzzle, and you know there is a solution. Most of us won't rest until we know what that solution is. When we are attracted to someone and feel romantic feelings for that person, his or her body, particularly the sex organs—which are about the only things covered up these days—become the source of considerable mystery. Wrapped up in a sexy package, it is a mystery that few men, or women, can resist.

LINGERIE

In Los Angeles, where I live, there are a number of lingerie shops, some of which actually put on shows and encourage couples to come in together. In some shops, the sales staff actually model the merchandise, and women are encouraged to try on lingerie. A man accompanying his girlfriend can appreciate the various outfits as they actually look on her, in the intimacy of a cozy dressing room. All in all, shopping for

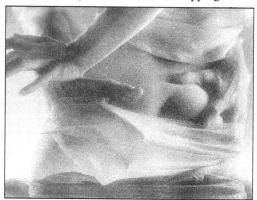

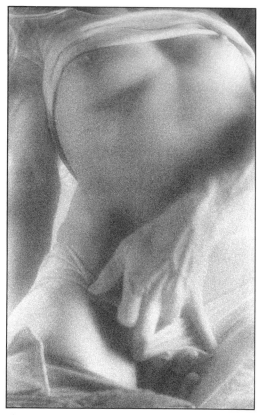

lingerie can, in itself, be a real turn-on.

But you don't have to be that exotic. Just rely on some old standbys, the turn-ons that have worked over the years, and you may just find out why they have lasted so long. The story of John W. illustrates the point.

"My girlfriend and I could be considered children of the '60s in many ways, and throughout most of the '70s we lived in a cabin in Northern California with our two dogs. Our sex had always been good, but pretty predictable and uninventive.

"We moved to L.A. in the early '80s, and I worked as a freelance artist doing catalogue work. One of the catalogues I was commissioned to do involved some illustrations for a mail-order lingerie company. While working on some of the drawings for the catalogue, I envisioned, and even drew a likeness of, Karen modeling black stockings and a black garter belt. I'd never really pictured her that way before, and I knew that Karen had never gone in for that type of sexuality. She is a very

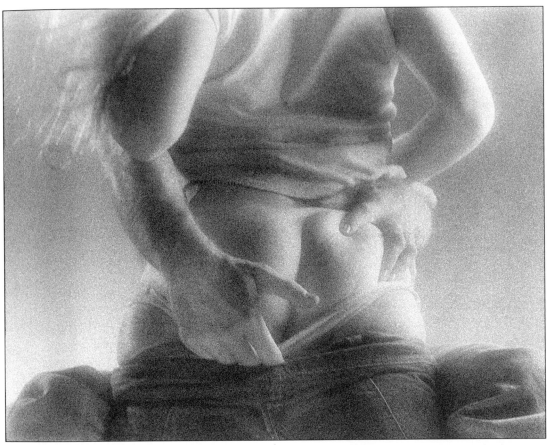

'earthy' sort of person.

"A couple of weeks later, I met with the owner of the lingerie company so he could approve my drawings. He liked them very much and, since we were meeting at his warehouse, he offered to let me take a few samples home to my girl-friend. At first, I said I'd pass. Then I remembered the stockings and garter belt, and I took him up on his offer.

"That night I showed Karen my drawings of her in the lingerie. and to my surprise she liked them very much. Then I brought out the stockings and garter belt. She was a little hesitant at first. To say this wasn't her thing is an under-statement. Even though she was an attractive woman, she usually wore practical, easy-on-the-feet natural shoes or thongs, jeans, and other 'pragmatic' clothing. She only owned one pair of high-heeled shoes, and she hadn't worn those in years.

"After some initial resistance, she dug out her high-heeled shoes and went into the bathroom to put on the garter belt and stockings. Mean-while, I went into the bedroom, lit some can-dles, and prepared the atmosphere. When she walked into the bedroom dressed in the stock-ings, garter belt, and high-heels, my heart skipped a beat. I can truthfully say that I've never seen a sexier-looking woman in the pages of any magazine than my Karen, the way she was dressed that night. It was a spectacular night in bed; I just could not get enough of her.

"Since then Karen has purchased lots of lingerie. In fact, after that night her whole wardrobe started to change, becoming more feminine. She now loves dressing up, saying it makes her feel more like a woman, and it has brought out a side of her that had been dor-mant all her adult life."

A WORD ABOUT ROMANCE

Whereas just meeting your lover in bed, naked,

as a matter of course before going to sleep can be satisfying and is often the most practical thing to do, it is usually not very romantic. Romance plays a larger part in the longevity of a relationship than does sex. As we all know, the unenhanced sex act seems to wane in intensity with time and familiarity. When it does occasionally rise again in intensity, it is usually because it is coupled with unusually strong feelings by the participants for each other.

Romance is a very misunderstood subject. One need look no further than TV, movies, or the bookstore to see how highly women value romance. It is generally the man who takes the blame for killing romance. All a man wants is sex, many a woman has been heard to complain. Although there is a grain—or two—of truth to that statement, I believe that men in fact want romance almost as much as women do. Every man has experienced the difference between having sex with a woman and making *love* with a woman. The actions may be the same—in fact, they may have taken place with the same woman. I have had the telling experience of having sex with a woman, then later, after becoming romantically involved with her, making love with her. The same act, the same moving parts, the same people, but the experiences were as different as night and day. In the latter case, we were in love, romantically involved, and the experience was much more satisfying.

The sex act itself may stay pretty much constant, but it's the feeling behind it that gives it the juice, makes it special or plain. The easiest way to revive a sagging sex life is to revive the couple's feelings for each other.

Don't forget what we've discussed regarding attitude, mood, and setting. More stages have been set by a bouquet of flowers than by all the stagehands on Broadway put together. Molly G. gives this advice to those who feel that their relationships are failing.

"Warren and I have been married for seventeen years. I know this may sound terribly old-fashioned, but when we got married we agreed that it would be forever and that, no matter what, we would never get a divorce. That doesn't mean we haven't had hard times that have mightily tried our resolve, yet we've never spoken of getting a divorce. It simply was not an option.

"Two things that have worked best for us over the years is a good, steady sex life and staying romantically involved with each other.

"One exercise that has worked like a charm with us is this. Whenever we're going through a tough period—when we're fighting a lot or we're just not in touch—we each go off in separate parts of the house and write down a few things. First of all, we write down the things we really like about each other, the things that are really special. We do this because when we're going through difficult times, we're usually focusing on things we don't like about each other. Or maybe we're just not focusing on each other at all.

"Then we write down the last time we really felt romantically involved with each other, and why. We try to write down all the feelings and reasons, so as to recall totally the feeling of being in love with each other. And usually the things we write down aren't what you might think. It usually isn't anything like candlelight dinners or wild weekends. I remember that the last time we did this I recalled a time when I came across a photograph of Warren smiling, sitting on the patio of a cabin we'd rented a few summers before in Lake Arrowhead. He didn't look particularly sexy or even well dressed. His hair was messed up, and he was wearing a T-shirt I'd bought him that afternoon. But there was something about him that was captured in the photograph. There was no one in the world like Warren, and in that photograph I saw something that was so sweet, innocent, and very, very loving. That he was my husband and willing to hang in there during times that I knew were just as tough for him as they were for me made me love him even more.

"After I recalled that incident, I went into the den where Warren was working on his list. Apparently he'd come up with something, too, because when I came in he turned toward me. In his face I could see only love where indifference and frustration were settling in quite comfortably only hours before. That night, as we do many nights when we perform our little exercise, we made passionate love, using sex the way the 'manufacturer' probably would have recommended had he been given the opportunity to put it on the label."

FOREPLAY

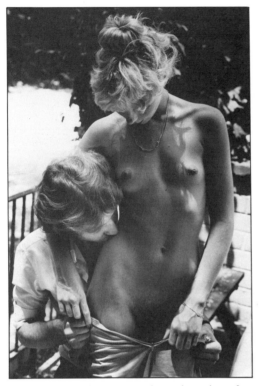

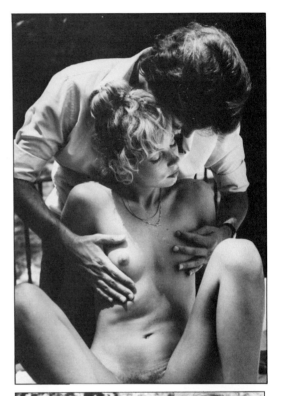

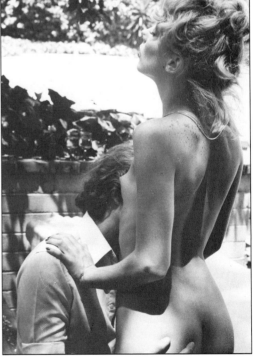

Foreplay is, basically, sex prior to insertion of the penis. In fact, it's difficult to pinpoint exactly where foreplay ends and "sex" begins. To illustrate, I recall dating a young woman in San Francisco whose boyfriend was out of town at the time. After engaging in considerable foreplay and an abundance of oral sex, I attempted to insert my penis into her vagina. She pulled back in horror, shook her head, and pushed me away. When I inquired why she was acting so strangely, she replied with a straight face that she had promised her boyfriend she wouldn't have sex with anyone while he was gone. This woman apparently had an extremely narrow view of what it meant to "have sex" with someone. Had her boyfriend walked in on us while she was giving me head, I doubt quite seriously if he would have agreed with her definition.

Foreplay is like the first act in the play of love. Some people, particularly women, complain that they usually don't get seated until the second act—wherein penis meets vulva, penis gets vulva, penis loses vulva.

There are many reasons why foreplay is overlooked. One is ignorance. Many men don't

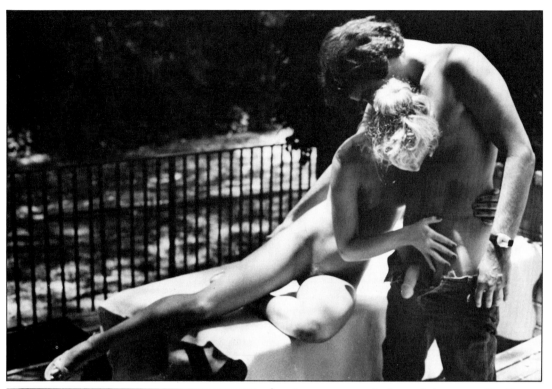

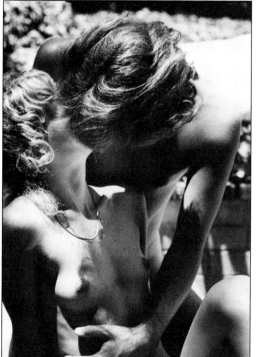

know very much about their partners' bodies and therefore either fumble or otherwise perform clumsily and ineffectively. A little communication could go a long way toward solving this problem.

MASTURBATION: DEMONSTRATING THE OBVIOUS

One obvious but little practiced method of educating a lover, male or female, is to have your partner watch you masturbate. Who knows your body better? You wrote the owner's manual for your body. If you're going to let somebody else drive it, he or she might as well know how it works. Watching each other masturbate can be a real turn-on for both parties. Don't be afraid to point out things that you're doing to yourself, as you're doing them, so your partner can really see what makes you feel good. Feel free to offer a hands-on demonstration, just to make sure your pupil is getting the hang of it.

Another reason men skim so glibly over foreplay is because they are too concerned with their own erection. In particular, they are concerned that once they've got it, they might lose

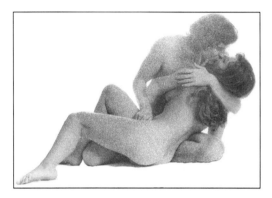

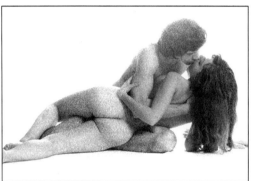

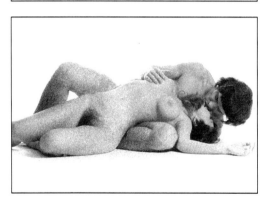

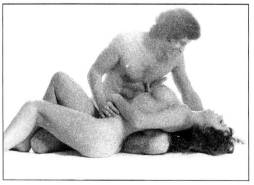

it. They seem to want to "hand it in" like a class project they're proud of and eager to present. The more insecure a man feels about his erection, the more likely he will be to remove foreplay from his sexual routine.

Experience and confidence can overcome such insecurities, and a man's partner can help considerably in this regard. If a woman enjoys foreplay, she can logically assume that her man enjoys it, too. Therefore, a woman should try to be aware of the man's needs and help him "set the table." One way of doing this is to caress his penis while the man is caressing her body. She should be aware that the penis is getting harder. She may choose to touch it, squeeze it, whatever, but the important thing is to stay in contact with it. One reason an insecure man may wish to enter his lover too soon is to prove to her that he can get a good erection. If his lover is in contact with his penis throughout foreplay, then he already knows that *she* knows his penis is hard. Therefore, the man no longer has to "prove himself."

Another reason a man may wish to skip foreplay is simply because he cares only about his own pleasure. Although some women may find this practice in itself somewhat erotic, they usually tire of it as a steady, never-changing diet.

TOUCHING
Most people are aware of the major erogenous zones, or areas of the body that are particularly sensitive to touch: they include the ears, mouth, forehead, nipples, toes, and almost every inch of skin below the navel and above the knees.

When someone says the word "touching," most people automatically think of touching with the hands or fingers. However, there are many other methods of touching. You can touch your lover with your lips, tongue, hair, toes, or any other part of your body. The next time you want to try something a little different, give your lover a sexy massage as a prelude to lovemaking. One of the sexiest massages I ever received was from a woman who had fairly long, silky hair. She hardly touched me with her fingers, but rather caressed me with her beautiful hair. Not only did she run it gently along my body, she also curled it around my penis. As she slowly raised her head, the hair sensuously unwrapped itself.

THE BREAST

Foreplay is any form of caressing that is used to get from not being totally ready to make love, to being ready. It would be difficult to find a better bridge between those two states, in terms of female arousal, than the breasts. When the nipples are caressed, the female sexual nerve network swings into high gear. Messages are sent to the sex organs that cause lubricants to prepare the vagina for sex. The clitoris begins to become erect.

A man can rarely go wrong by spending a portion of his foreplay time caressing, licking, and/or sucking the breasts. Some women like the feel of a man "biting" their nipples. Naturally, care should be taken not to bite too hard.

Certainly men respond to the sight of breasts. *Playboy* built an empire exposing them. Why men enjoy them so much is hard to say. Someone could write an entire book on the psychology of why men love breasts, but that isn't as important as simply knowing that this is true.

Oral sex will be covered in greater detail later in the book. However, a word about it here seems appropriate. Many men enjoy having fellatio performed on them by their lovers during foreplay. There are several reasons for this. First, it's an almost foolproof method for attaining a good erection. Second, most men find it visually stimulating to see their partners giving them head. Women enjoy this practice also and get to feel the penis swell from its limp state to a rockhard readiness in their mouths.

Cunnilingus is also a useful foreplay tool. At least that's the way Terry S. sees it.

"My wife, Gloria, and I always had a decent sex life—not bad, but nothing to write home about, if you know what I mean. She's about five years younger than I am, and when we first got together she was 19. One thing that became obvious very fast was that I liked to have sex a lot more than she did. I enjoyed having sex about five times a week and she was quite happy with just once or twice a week.

"Once she got going, she was a real tiger in bed, but getting her in the mood was a real problem. Usually when we went to bed, she said she was too tired and would gently but firmly repel all my advances. We'd been married about a year, and I was really frustrated about what I considered to be my wife's lack of sexual desire.

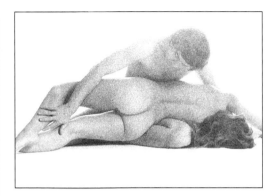

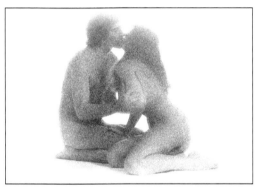

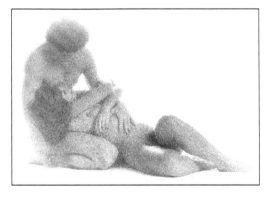

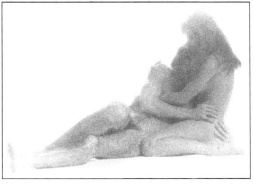

FOREPLAY

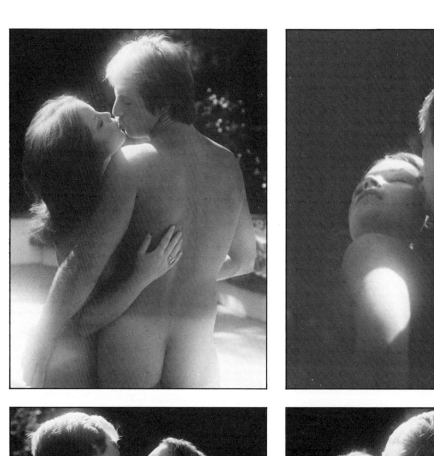

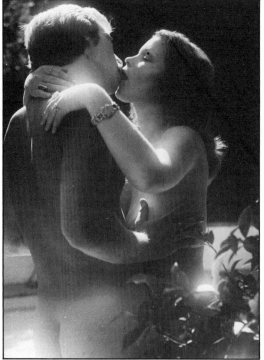

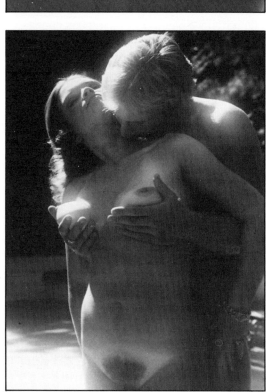

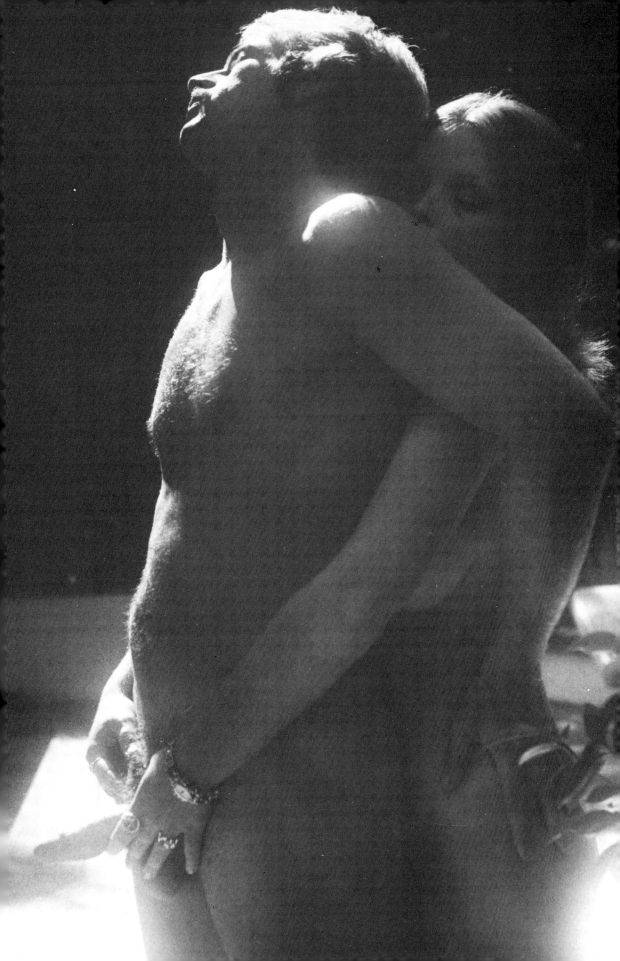

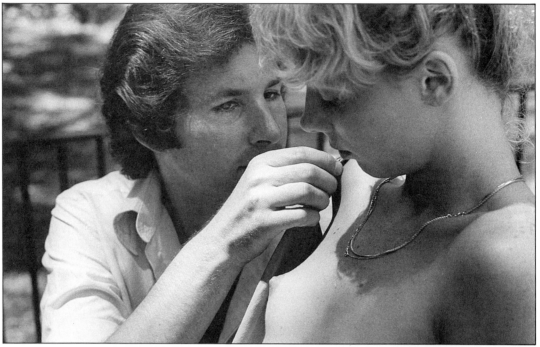

Eventually, I reached the end of my rope.

"I'd recently discovered that Gloria really enjoyed cunnilingus—especially performed the way I'd read about it being done in a book a friend gave me. I'd never started our lovemaking sessions with cunnilingus before. Usually, whenever I did it—which wasn't too often—it was after we'd been making love for a while.

"One night I decided to take drastic measures. Up until this time I had always been quite the gentleman and deferred whenever Gloria gave the slightest indication that she wasn't in the mood. It was a hot summer night, and we were sleeping nude without any covers on. Tonight, as she lay sleeping soundly, I slid down and, slowly at first, started to flick her clitoris with my tongue. Gloria started to moan as she gradually came out of a deep sleep. By the time she was fully awake, she was screaming for me to get inside her. Naturally, I was glad to oblige.

"I decided to use cunnilingus as a form of foreplay again the next night—this time while Gloria was awake. After some very weak resistance—more out of habit than anything else—she let me go down on her, and again she ended up screaming for me to get inside her.

"Since then, cunnilingus has become a regu-

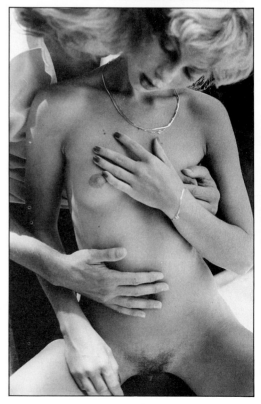

38

lar part of our foreplay. The key thing was, I simply found out what my wife liked and gave it to her."

Find out what someone likes and deliver it—sounds basic, doesn't it? Many times it's that simple.

KISSING

Remember kissing? Amazing as this may sound, many couples don't kiss. Or at least they don't kiss like they used to. If you're like most people,

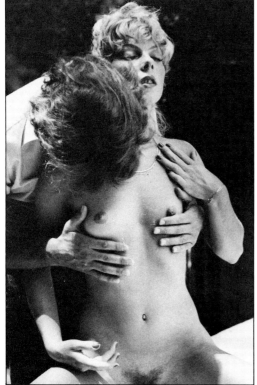

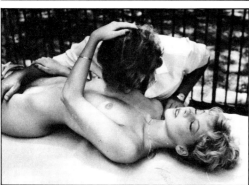

the kiss was probably the fuse that ignited most of the initial fires between you and your lover. As time goes on, however, the kiss is often relegated to perfunctory status.

But the kiss is such an intimate act. The next time you and your lover are getting your engines running, stay a little longer in first gear and explore each other's mouths, lips, and tongues.

THE RING GRIP

Many men enjoy a woman's aggressiveness dur-

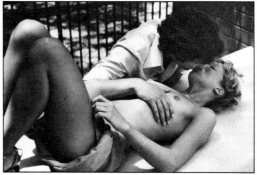

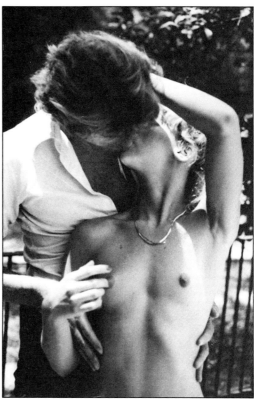

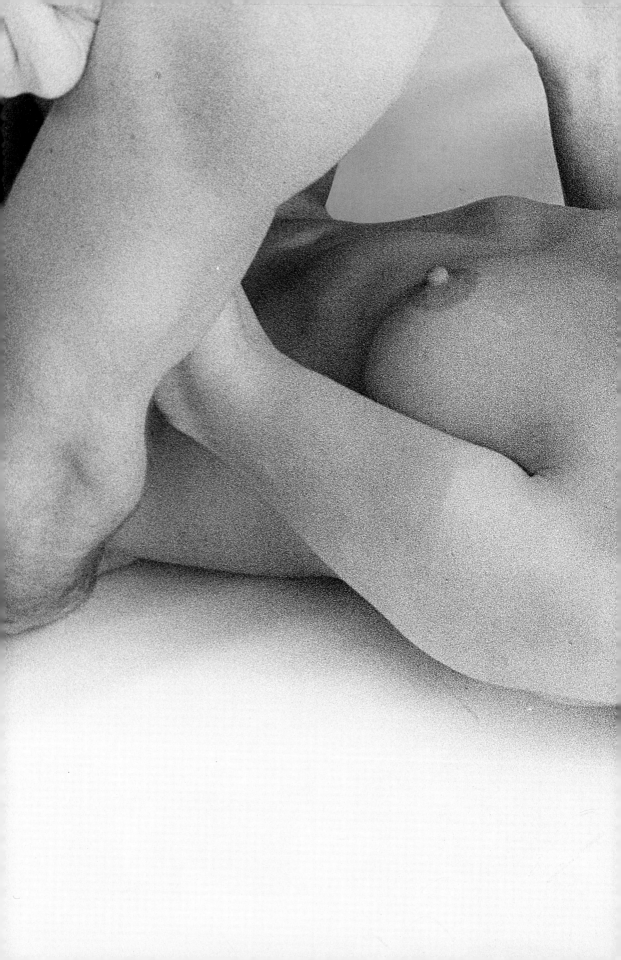

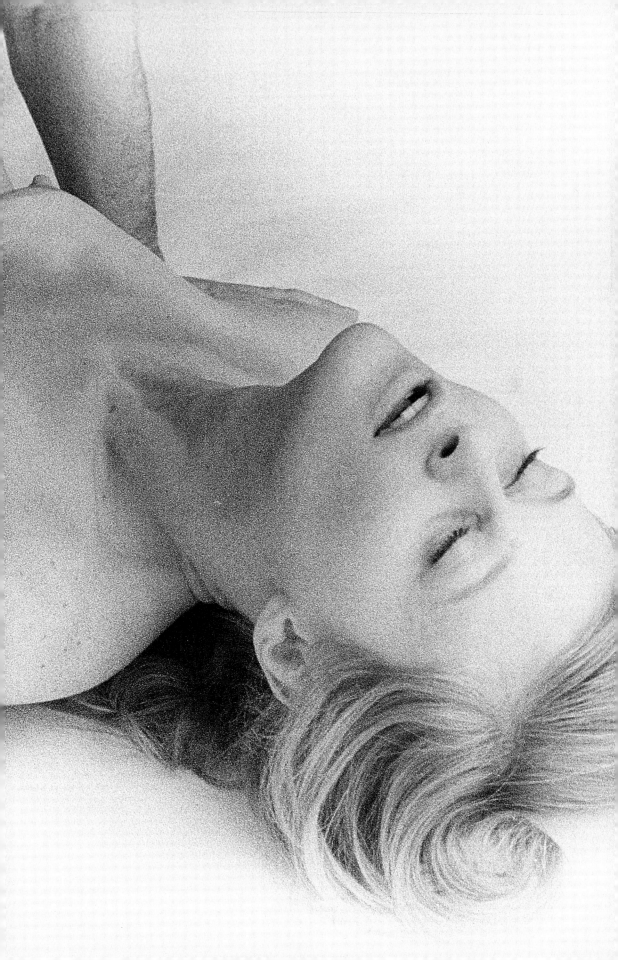

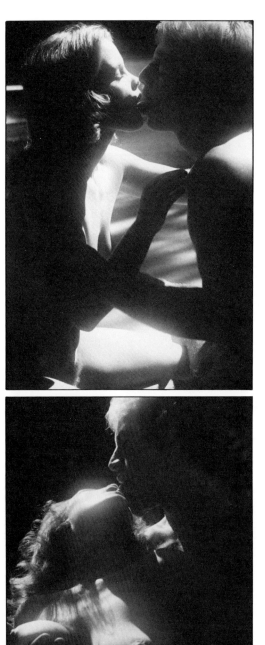
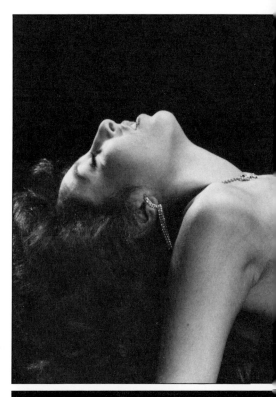
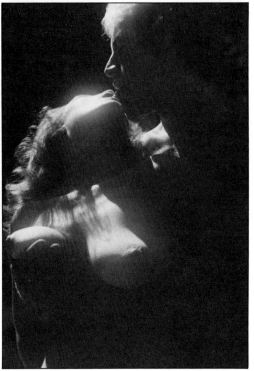
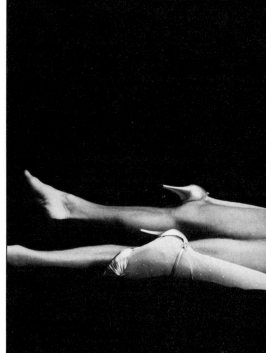

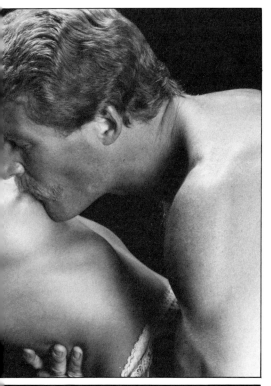

ing foreplay. One technique a woman should know if she is going to stimulate the penis is the "ring grip." It is actually quite simple. As the blood rushes into the penis and makes it erect, she can wrap her index finger and thumb around the base of the penis, thereby "locking" the blood supply in the penis. As she tightens this grip, the erection will increase. Alternately squeezing and releasing this grip can be quite exciting and stimulating to the man—and to his partner as well.

MONITORING THE WOMAN'S SEXUAL READINESS

It is easy to tell when the man is ready to move from foreplay to intercourse, but it is not as easy to tell when a woman is ready. Although she may be ready mentally and emotionally, a woman's body will sometimes take a little time to become lubricated and ready for her partner to enter.

It is a good idea for the man to stay in touch with his partner's vulva. A simple scenario for enjoyable foreplay that also allows the man to monitor his partner's readiness is as follows. With the woman lying on her back, her legs

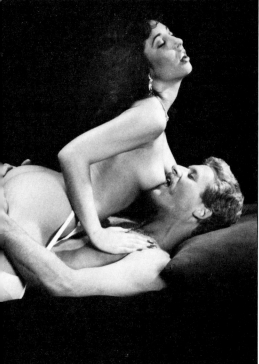

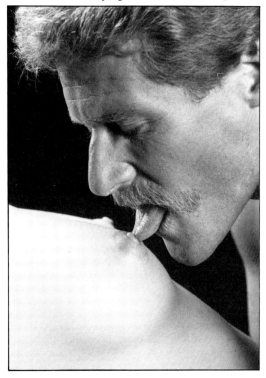

spread slightly, the man lies on his side parallel to his lover. In this position, he may kiss or lick her lips, neck, ears, nipples, etc. Meanwhile, with his hand he can stimulate the clitoris, vagina, and/or anus.

A "three-pronged" approach can produce a very pleasant response. With his thumb, the man can stimulate the clitoris, with his middle finger he can caress the vagina, and with his small or ring finger he can caress the anus or even insert his finger inside it. (NOTE: If you do insert a finger inside the anus, DO NOT put

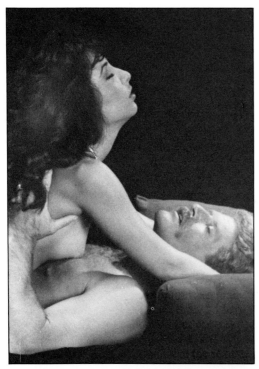

that finger inside the vagina, because this can cause a vaginal infection.) Instead of caressing the anus with the small or ring finger, a man may choose to caress the perineum.

While the man is stimulating his lover in this fashion, he is also able to rub his penis against his lover's thigh in order to maintain his erection.

This technique is perfect for foreplay not only because many women find it wildly exciting, but also because the man is able to stay in constant contact with the woman's vagina, thereby being able to determine when she is ready to be entered.

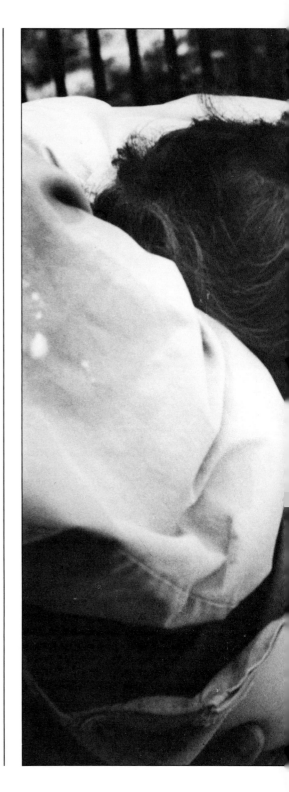

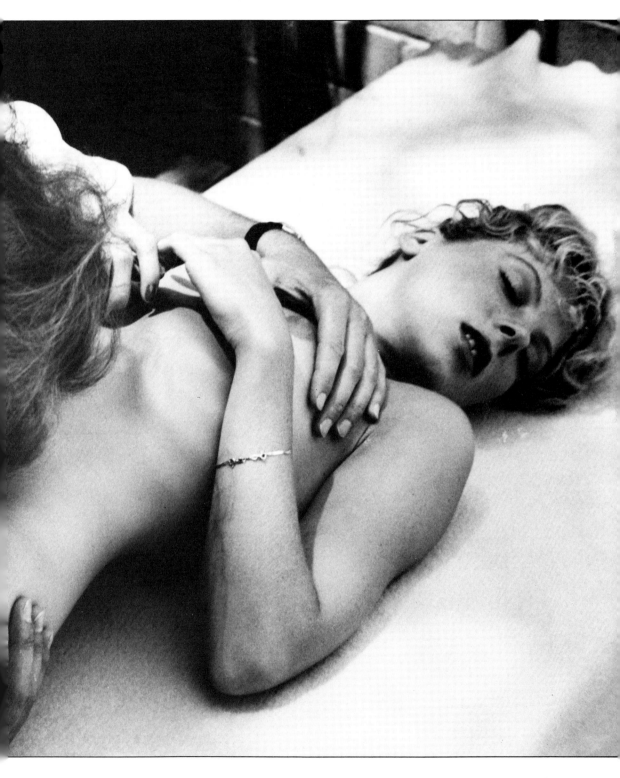

ORAL · SEX

It was not so very long ago that oral sex was on the list of offbeat sexual practices considered taboo. In fact, there are those among us who still, for one reason or another, consider oral sex to be a perversion. But then, there are still those among us who believe that Elvis is alive and living in Greece.

One thing that should be obvious, but worth mentioning because many obvious things escape our notice, is that hygiene plays an important role in one's enjoyment of oral sex. Good hygiene is an excellent habit to get into. It's a good idea to shower or at least clean the areas that will "see the most action," including the genitals and the anus (whether or not you in-

tend to bring the anus directly into play). Regardless of whether oral sex is contemplated, hygiene should be a regular part of your sexual regimen.

After washing, you may wish to accent your genital area or upper thighs with perfume or cologne. But be careful. You don't want to drown your genitals with fragrance, for at least two reasons. First, the smell of the genitals themselves, when clean and aroused, can be extremely stimulating (especially the female genitals, which secrete an abundance of fluids). Second, most perfumes and colognes contain alcohol and other substances that may not be pleasant to the taste when contacted directly by

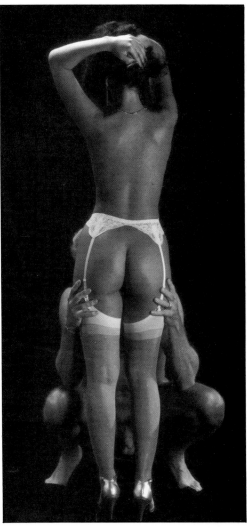

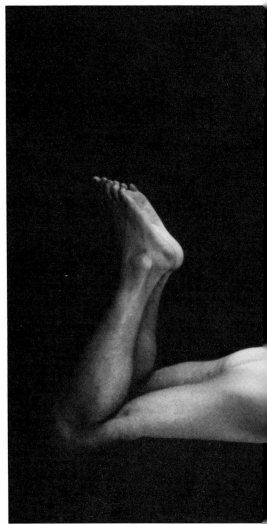

the tongue, and can serve as an irritant to the genitals themselves.

MAN TO WOMAN

If a man knows how to perform cunnilingus, he can almost always bring his partner to orgasm. In order to perform it correctly, the man must first know the component parts of the female genitalia. If you have read this book from the beginning, this should not be a problem. If you have just opened the book to this chapter, however, flip back to the illustration of the female genitalia (pg. 17) to familiarize yourself with basic anatomy.

A few comments are in order here regarding the classic "69" position, wherein couples are able to give each other oral stimulation simultaneously. From a practical point of view, this position is considerably overrated because it does not provide adequate access to the specific "trigger" points on the penis and clitoris that usually require stimulation in order to achieve orgasm. I'm not saying that it is impossible to achieve orgasm via the "69" position, only that it is demonstrably more difficult to do so than in other positions that provide ideal access to these points.

An ideal position in which to perform cunnilingus is for the woman to be flat on her back, knees lifted, feet flat on the bed. The man

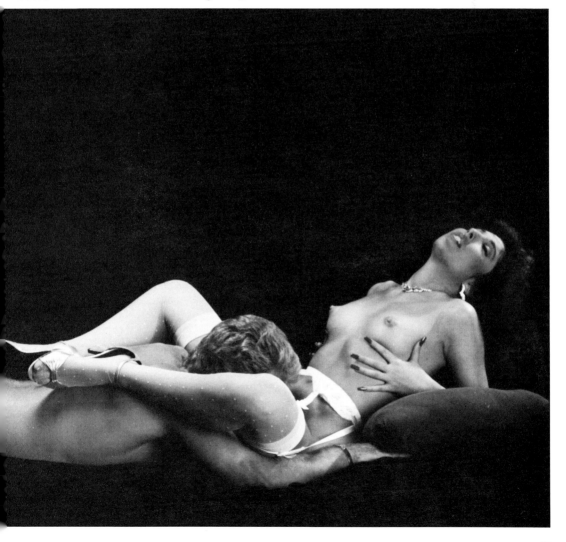

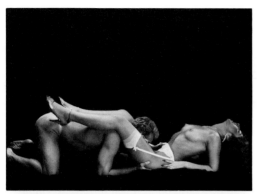

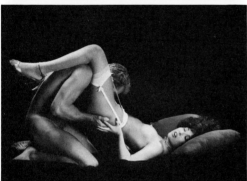

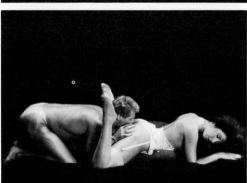

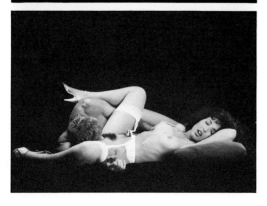

approaches from between her legs, facing the vulva. This position provides several distinct advantages. First, visually the man is able to see not only his partner's genitals, but also her stomach, breasts, and face. Second, his hands are free to stimulate the woman's genitals, breasts, anus, etc. Third, and most important, this position provides perfect access to the clitoris. With his tongue, the man can "scoop up" the clitoris, roll it around, flick it, tap it, lick it, or whatever else he may wish to do with it. While it is stimulating to the woman for the man to lick her labia and the entire vulva in general, the real target here is the clitoris.

As with all forms of lovemaking, once you know the basics, the best approach is often the creative one. Consider the experience of Ron H.

"I was never that much into oral sex until I started seeing my current girlfriend, Mary Ann. She's 21, five years younger than I am. One thing about Mary Ann is that she's clean—I mean, really clean. She must take a shower two or three times a day.

"I must have had a thing about giving head to my girlfriends before Mary Ann, because I just couldn't get very excited about it. I remember thinking in the back of my mind that there was something kind of demeaning about my giving some girl head. And it seemed so unsanitary. Both of these objections were overcome with Mary Ann, and I found myself interested in getting into oral sex with her more and more.

"One night, on her birthday, I decided to really give her a special treat. I knew she liked my giving her head, so I told her to relax and enjoy—that I was in control. I turned her over on her side, and lifted her upper leg so that it was almost drawn into her chest. I approached her, with my tongue, from behind, my feet up toward the back of her head. With her upper leg spread wide, I could see her squeaky-clean pussy and her even squeakier-clean anus. Licking someone's anus was one of those things I used to wince at whenever I heard of anyone doing it. But that night, as I looked at Mary Ann's anus, it just looked so sexy—and I knew it was clean. So I started gently licking her upper thighs and buttocks, getting closer and closer to her anus without touching it. Mary Ann was going wild in anticipation. When my tongue flicked across her asshole, I thought

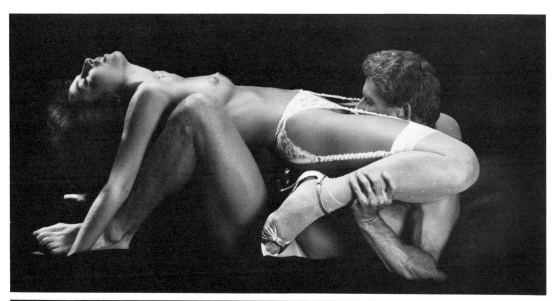

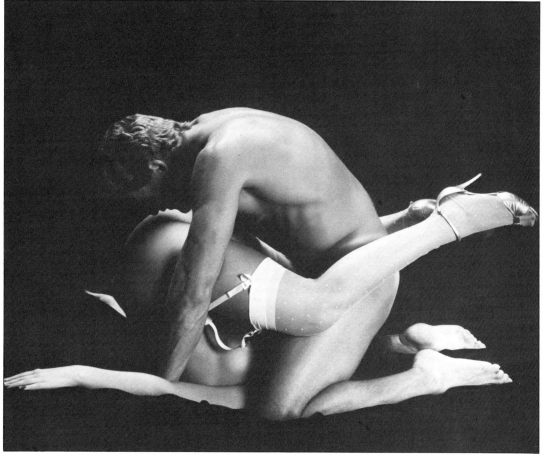

she was going to explode. But that was just the beginning.

"When I was finally willing to get down and look at Mary Ann's clit and her other genital anatomy up close, I have to admit that it really looked pretty to me. As I was tickling her clit with my tongue, I had an inspiration. I gently sucked her clit between my teeth, being careful not to bite down or scratch it, totally isolating it between my teeth. After that, I was able to flick, lick, or tongue-massage Mary Ann's clit with more control than I'd ever had before. She just about went out of her mind. She had an orgasm like I'd never seen her have before—like I've never seen, or heard, anyone have.

"I really enjoy giving Mary Ann head now, and naturally she loves it. I also enjoy the feeling of control I get by having my lover's 'pleasure center' in my mouth, knowing that I'm capable of making it explode any time I want to."

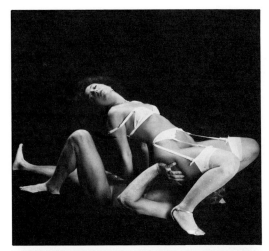

Orally exploring your partner can be quite an adventure. Besides being fun, it can provide an education in what makes your lover tick, sexually. See how he or she responds to different stimuli. Does she like a caress better than a bite? Or does a bite really get her motor running? A bite where? Does she like lots of stimulation on her vulva, and less on her breasts? Or does she like it the other way around? You can learn a lot from this sort of experimentation that can give you ideas for other positions or fantasies that she might enjoy, based on what

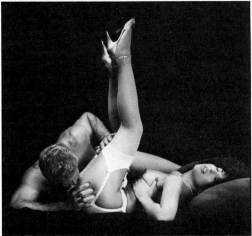

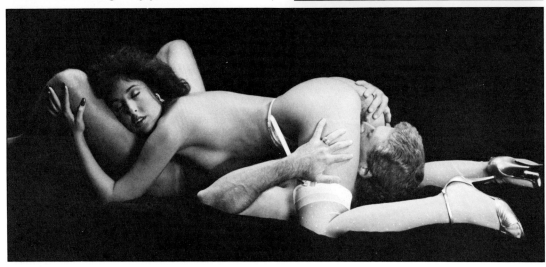

you've discovered orally.

And don't forget the other erogenous zones, including ears, lips, breasts, and thighs. Your mouth can do things to a nipple that your fingers cannot do. It can suck, lick, bite, and blow warm or cool air, producing an exciting variety of sensations and combinations.

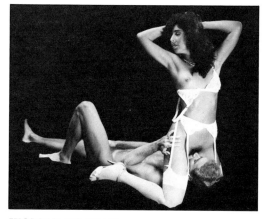

WOMAN TO MAN

Since I have repeatedly made the point in this book that people are generally uninformed or misinformed about sex, it should come as no great surprise that many women don't know how to perform fellatio. Never is this more evident than when a woman approaches a man from above, as in the "69" position, and tries to bring him to climax by frantically licking the topmost surface of his penis. Not only will this usually not work, it can be extremely irritating.

(Orgasms can result from this position, however, from indirect friction applied to the correct spot, which is under the penis.)

The proper way to give head is to stimulate the spot on the underside of the penis where the head, or ring, is joined to the shaft. Therefore, the best position is for the woman to approach the man in a manner similar to the one described above for man-to-woman oral sex. That is, the man lies on his back, legs spread apart, and the woman, on her knees or stomach, takes his penis in her mouth, licking the underside of the penis as she slides her head up and down along the shaft, occasionally sucking the penis. She may also choose to lay the penis back on the man's stomach and lick or flick along the underside of the shaft as the penis grows more and more rigid.

Once the penis starts to get hard, a woman may wish to slide her hand up and down as she takes the penis in and out of her mouth. Lubrication should not be a problem at this point because the woman's saliva should be covering the penis by this time. Orgasm can be easily achieved by performing fellatio in this manner.

When orgasm is achieved, what do you do with the semen? This is a personal choice. Some women will never get used to the idea of swallowing semen. Others can't get enough of it, preferring to lick it off their lovers' cocks after any type of orgasm. The myths about semen being harmful to swallow are false, as should be self-evident to any clear-thinking person.

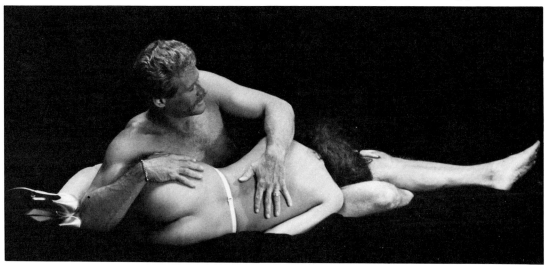

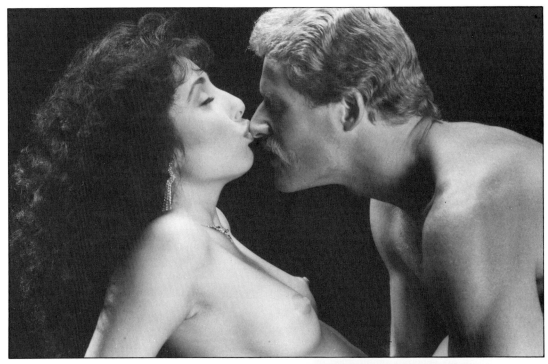

Many men find it quite exciting to see a woman swallow their semen. However, if the woman chooses not to swallow it, she should have a tissue or towel handy in order to dispose of the semen. Otherwise, the sight of the woman leaping out of bed and racing to the bathroom to "spit up" puts a definite damper on the mood, which should be warm and comforting after sex.

The woman should also take care that her teeth do not scratch her partner's penis. It happens all the time, but for some reason, unless it's severe, many men feel awkward about telling their lovers that they are doing something wrong. Speaking up, however, may prove deeply gratifying—as Paul T. discovered.

"I really love my wife, Christy, but when we first got together, having her give me head was a nightmare. She really had no idea of what to do. She was always licking the wrong side of my penis and mistaking my cries of agony for cries of pleasure, which just made her lick harder and harder. On top of that, it was like putting my cock into a meat grinder, because when she wasn't licking me the wrong way, she was bouncing her head up and down on my

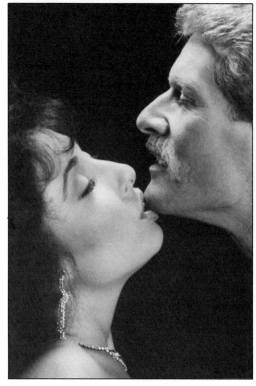

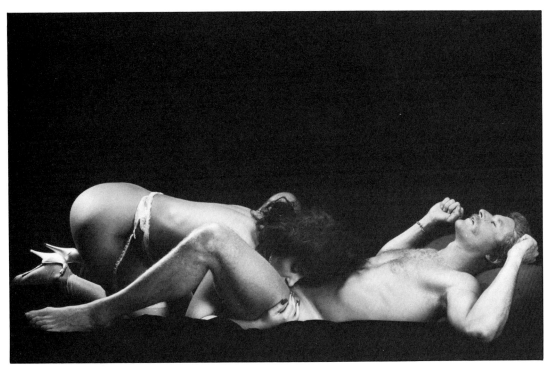

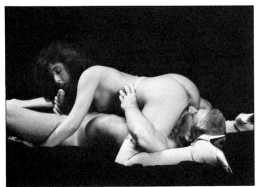

cock and not opening her mouth enough. This led to her teeth scratching the sensitive skin of my penis.

"Finally I couldn't take it any longer. In the most loving way possible, I told her that I didn't want her to give me head again until she learned how to do it. At first she was a little hurt, but she finally took it in the spirit I'd intended and actually seemed to welcome the challenge.

"We didn't talk about it for a month or so after that. Then one night while we were making love, she went down on me. I could hardly believe I was with the same woman. It was as though her tongue could read my body. She flicked her tongue all along the underside of my penis, then tickled my anus with her tongue. When I was almost ready to come, she stopped me by taking my penis out of her mouth and knowledgeably wrapping her fingers around the base. 'No you don't,' she said. 'I want you to shoot it way down my throat.'

"I wasn't sure exactly what she was talking about, but by now I was more than willing to follow her anywhere. She lay down on her back across the bed, so that her head was hanging over the edge. Then she motioned me over until I was standing above her open mouth. I positioned myself on the edge of the bed so as to provide myself the best access to her waiting mouth. The tilt of her head backward made it possible for me to insert my penis all the way into her throat. She lay perfectly still as I used her mouth and throat, and when I came, the force was like a hurricane.

"Later, while we were cuddling in bed, I asked her what she had done to become so good at giving head. She said that she'd read a book on oral sex that her girlfriend had

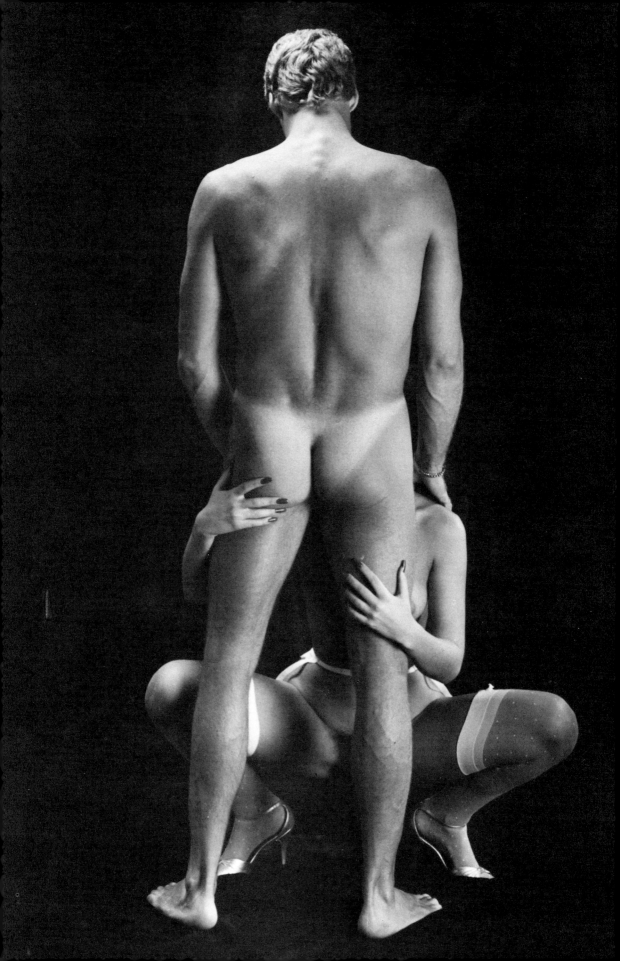

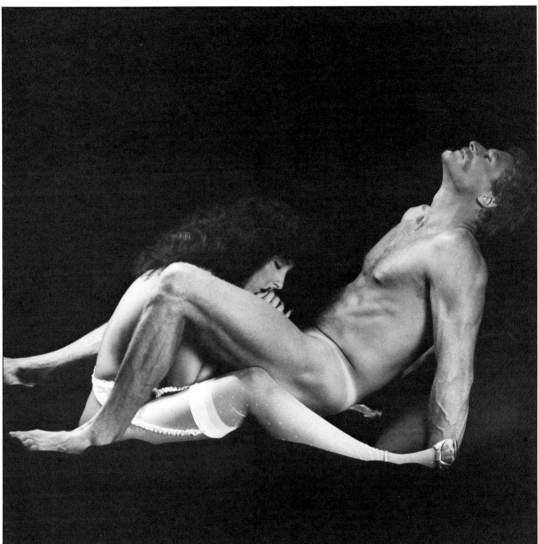

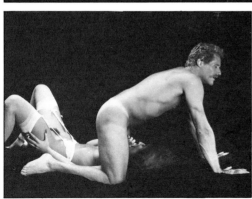

recommended. *As for the 'deep-throating' ability, she said she'd used a carrot to practice with.*

"This may sound silly, but I was proud of Christy for having thought enough of our relationship and my desires to take the time to go out and learn something that would make me happy."

I'm not sure I would have bought the story about the carrot. Nonetheless, this story proves that even though people have been making love for some time, they can, through communication and education, learn new techniques that can dramatically improve their relationship.

ORGASM

DELAYED OR NON-ORGASM-ORIENTED INTERCOURSE

Who among us can deny that we are an orgasm-oriented people? The evidence is overwhelming. Barbara, a distraught friend of mine, related this telling story to me over a couple of vodkas not long ago.

"Things aren't going so well between Bill and me these days. In fact, I'm thinking of leaving him."

"What's the problem?" I inquired. "I thought things were really great between you two."

"They were. But . . ."

"You can tell me," I said. "We were friends long before you met Bill. What's the problem?"

She hesitated, then said, "It's quite personal. I hope this doesn't make you feel any differently toward Bill."

I assured her that it would not.

"All right, I'll tell you. Bill can only give me one orgasm when we make love."

While that revelation truly didn't make me feel any differently toward Bill, it did make me think that my friend Barbara might have recently lost her citizenship in the land of the quick.

"Barbara," I began, "what makes you think that's bad?"

She recited quotes from several articles she'd read in the past few months, plus "information" from a friend of hers who had assured her that "everyone" who was anyone was having orgasms in the double and triple-digit range—if they were with a compatible partner.

I suggested a couple of other articles she might read and gave her a few books. I also assuerd her that many women would envy her the fact that she was able to achieve a predictable, good orgasm every time she made love.

This is an interesting and true story, but it doesn't even begin to take into consideration the real issue. And that is, are we so orgasm-oriented that we forget about love? Put another way, even if we are sensation-oriented, aren't we missing the bulk of the sensations available from lovemaking if we focus our attention solely upon orgasm? It's much like driving from New York to Los Angeles and sleeping from city limit to city limit. You miss the journey. What happens on the journey from foreplay to orgasm is where the heart of the matter, the substance, is to be found.

Usually the purpose of making love with someone is to give sensation and to experience sensation. And most of the sensations occur during lovemaking long before orgasm is achieved.

Recently I spoke with a friend of mine whom I hadn't seen since college. I told him about the book I was writing, and he told me this story.

"When I first met my wife, Gina, she was teaching yoga at a local health club. I started taking classes from her, and eventually we started dating. I had taken several philosophy classes in college and had a real interest in Eastern philosophy. One night while browsing through Gina's books, I came across a volume on Tantric Yoga, or sexual yoga. I borrowed the book and read it.

"Initially I was quite skeptical, because one of the major premises in the book was that a man should try to hold or retain his orgasm. Among the reasons given were that it was more healthful to retain the sexual energy and circulate it throughout the body, and that orgasm depleted men of vital fluids and energy necessary for good health and mental sharpness.

"Even though I had my reservations, I decided to try holding back my orgasm the next time Gina and I made love. Several interesting things happened when I did this. First, we made love for a much longer time than usual. Second, I felt closer to her than usual. Like seeing a house for the first time, even though you drive by it every day, I saw Gina physically, spiritually, and emotionally as I had never seen her before. Third, when we got out of bed, I was even more full of energy than when we'd started to make love—usually I took a short nap after I had an orgasm. Fourth, my feelings for Gina seemed to carry over from our lovemaking session right on through to all of our other activities, even though we were no longer 'making love.' I looked at her differently, almost as though we were still making love even though I wasn't inside her.

"Since then—and that was about two years ago—we have continued this practice. I occasionally have orgasms, but not more than a couple of times a month. Interestingly, however, Gina and I make love more often—at least once a night—than we did before."

Sometimes even though a man may wish to retain his ejaculation, a woman may demand

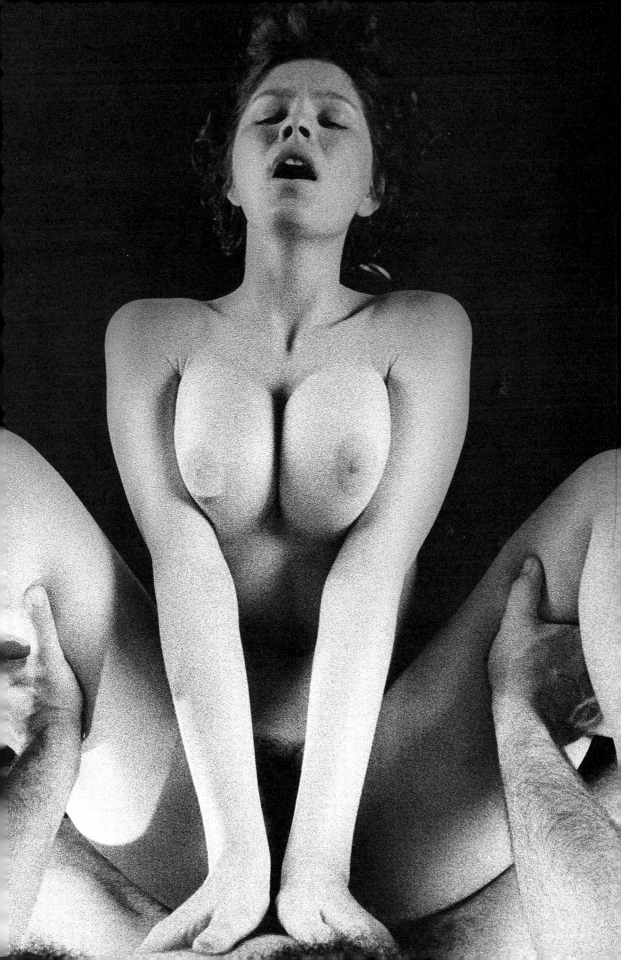

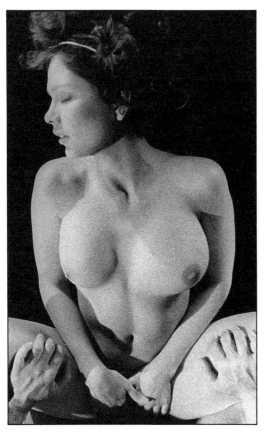 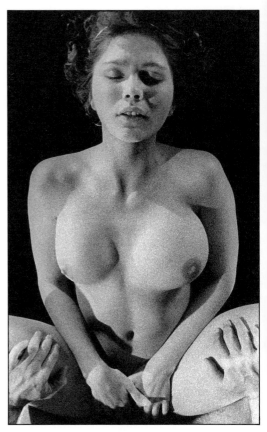

that he come inside her, saying that she will not be satisfied unless he does so. However, this "need" is more psychological than physiological and can usually be handled by the man reassuring his lover that he is completely satisfied by other sensations and pleasures he experiences while making love with her, and not simply by ejaculating inside her. Also, when the woman experiences greater sensation, warmth, and caring through prolonged, more knowing, and confident lovemaking, a gradual understanding and acceptance will occur naturally.

Doctors in the Orient, particularly practitioners of acupuncture, extol the virtues of retaining male fluids. According to their doctrines, considerable health and healing power abides in the semen and sperm. In fact, some Chinese literature recommends that young men ejaculate no more than twice a week. Middle-aged men are discouraged from ejaculating more than twice a month, and men over fifty are warned not to emit their seminal fluid at all. Depending on

what book you're reading, you may be advised to withhold ejaculation for a number of strokes (up to several thousand), for a period of hours, days, or months, or to abstain from ejaculation altogether.

Regardless of what the specific recommendation may be, all these suggestions reflect a single theme: controlling ejaculation will result in physiological, psychological, and emotional benefits for the man who has the patience to do so. Whereas most men would guard their right to orgasm as sacred and would pout mightily for days if it were taken away from them, it would be difficult to find a man who has not experienced, maybe without even being aware of them, the negative side effects of too many orgasms.

The most common manifestation is extreme drowsiness immediately following orgasm. Note that this fatigue does not necessarily follow prolonged sexual activity, but it does immediately follow orgasm, even if the sexual activity lasted

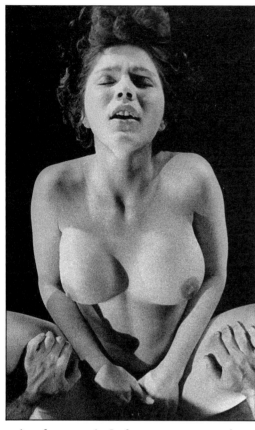
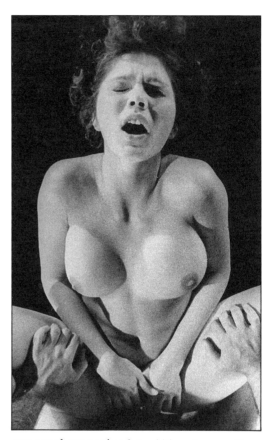

only a few seconds. In fact, a common routine for many couples is to make love just before going to sleep. Most men will tell you that after making love and ejaculating a considerable number of times in a relatively short span of time, they feel markedly more tired than usual. They may say this with a macho wink, but nonetheless they are experiencing a definite fatigue brought on by too many ejaculations in too short an amount of time. If a man were performing almost any other type of activity that caused such fatigue, he would moderate or suspend that activity immediately.

EJACULATION CONTROL
The easiest way to control your ejaculation, of course, is not to have sex, but such a policy deals a serious blow to optimum sexual relations with your partner.

The most obvious method of controlling ejaculation, short of abstinence, is to withdraw the penis for several seconds when you feel that you are about to ejaculate. Although you will lose a small percentage of your erection, after the wave of climax passes you will immediately be able to resume intercourse and your erection can be "rebuilt." The key here is to recognize an imminent ejaculation in time to stop it before it's too late. This just takes practice.

Another method of controlling ejaculation is to place the middle and forefinger of one hand between the scrotum and the anus when you recognize that ejaculation is near, and press. Some Chinese practitioners also recommend that the man take a deep breath at the same time. This method has several advantages. First, withdrawal of the penis is not required, so that intercourse is not interrupted. Second, it is not necessary to communicate what is happening to your partner. Even if you are not interested in retaining an orgasm indefinitely, this method of control is excellent for anyone who wishes to prolong sexual activity, including the man with a tendency toward premature ejaculation.

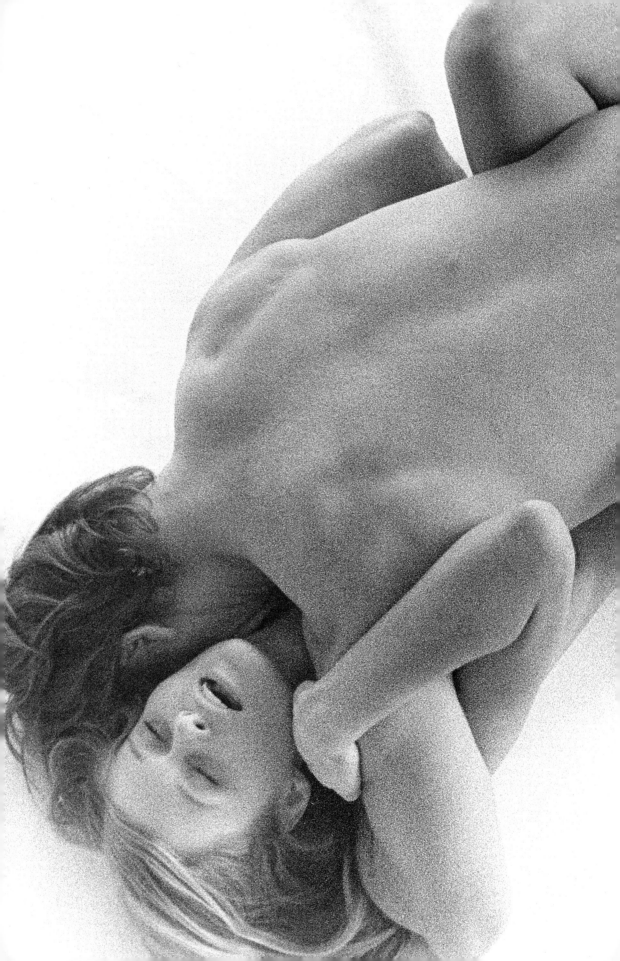

THE GRAFENBERG ORGASM

Female orgasm is almost as controversial a subject as penis size. In some male-oriented cultures, female satisfaction has been downplayed and knowledge about the female orgasm hidden even deeper than other information about sex. With the rising demands for female equality in recent times, however, has come the demand for equality in the orgasm department.

As with many injustices when they are righted, women's demand for orgasmic parity has at times gone a little overboard. Some women, previously quite satisfied with their love lives with their husbands or boyfriends, now read an article or catch an interview on TV and all of a sudden "realize" that they are not *really* being satisfied after all.

Although there is a legitimate point to be made by many women who want their mates to become more knowledgeable of female anatomy—their own, that is—there is sometimes an unfortunate tendency to turn the whole matter into a numbers game. There is no set number of orgasms per session, per hour, per week, or per relationship that will satisfy all women. Each woman is different. Some women will be able to achieve orgasm only with a partner for whom she has deep emotional feelings. Some women can achieve orgasm simply by crossing their legs.

Many women find it easier to achieve clitoral orgasms than vaginal ones. Clitoral orgasms are basically the same orgasm a woman achieves when she masturbates, except that instead of her fingers rubbing against the clitoris, it may be her lover's penis or pubic bone.

Women are also capable of achieving vaginal orgasms, as well as a combination of vaginal and clitoral orgasms at the same time, or during the same lovemaking session.

Recently there has been considerable talk and speculation about a specific spot inside the vagina which, when stimulated, will produce an orgasm. That spot has been called the Grafenberg Spot, and the resultant orgasm, the Grafenberg Orgasm.

The first step toward achieving the Grafenberg Orgasm is to locate your own Grafenberg Spot. When you're aroused (or even after you've come), put a finger in the vagina—your middle finger because it's the longest—and locate the

reference points on the upper (forward) surface of the vaginal wall (see diagram). First, locate the lumpy Skene's gland just inside the opening. Second, locate the hard area that you can feel through the skin (that's the corner of the pubic bone). Third, locate the smooth area leading back to the cervix (which you may or may not be able to reach, depending on the length of your finger). Now come back to the pubic bone with your finger and, hooking the finger in back of it, find a little hollow just before the smooth area begins. Your finger will be pointing

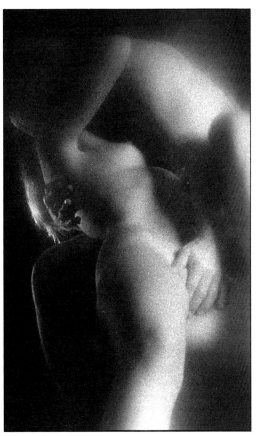

up toward your navel at this point, not back toward the cervix and the anus.

Probe this region firmly with your finger. When you touch the Grafenberg Spot, you'll feel a jolt and a momentary urge to urinate. If that feeling alarms you, you may want to quit at this point—but don't. Many women miss extra sexual pleasure because the association between sexual arousal and possible urinary incontinence

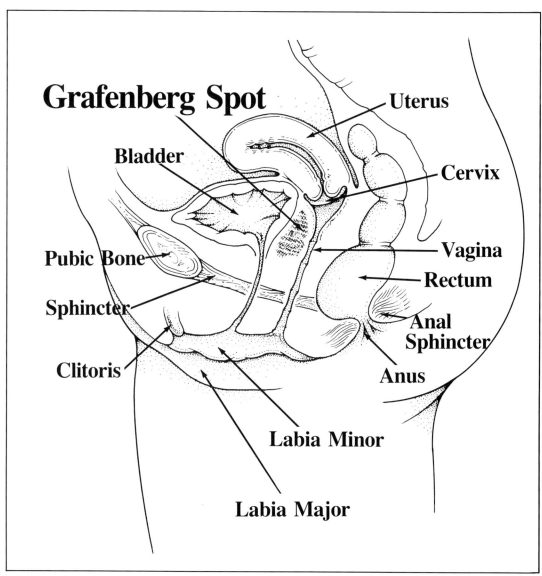

Grafenberg Spot

Uterus

Bladder

Cervix

Pubic Bone

Vagina

Sphincter

Rectum

Anal Sphincter

Clitoris

Anus

Labia Minor

Labia Major

makes them feel uneasy. If you are one of these women, simply empty your bladder and try again. Without this concern, you are free to stroke the Grafenberg Spot (which in many cases will swell and harden until it feels like a small bean under the surface of the skin) until the urgency to urinate passes and turns into a warm, deep, sensual feeling that is distinctly different from clitoral stimulation. You can sometimes intensify the feeling by pushing on the corresponding area of the lower abdomen while stimulating the spot from inside.

Whereas a clitoral orgasm feels sudden, sharp, and explosive, with its sensation limited to the pelvic area and very narrowly focused, the Grafenberg Orgasm appears to be deeper, slower, more relaxed, bathing the whole body in a warm, wavelike spread of sensation.

The best positions for the penis to make contact with the Grafenberg Spot usually involve the man entering the vagina from behind. Also, the woman-on-top positions allow the woman to manipulate the penis so that it contacts the Grafenberg Spot.

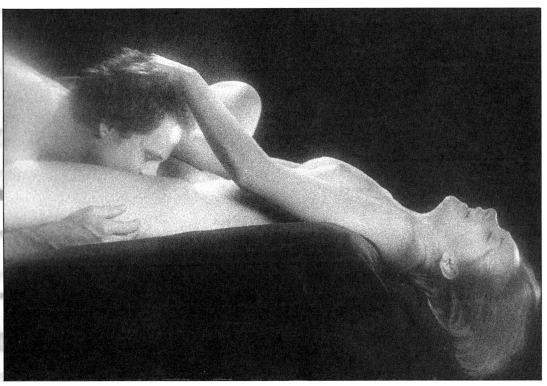

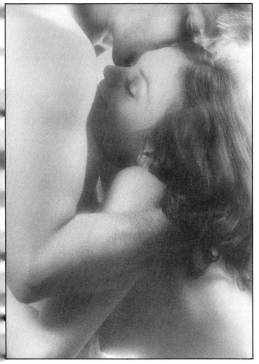

It is extremely helpful for the woman to educate her lover regarding the Grafenberg Spot. This can be done easily by performing the aforementioned location exercise with your lover's finger instead of your own. Once he and you both know exactly where it is, it will be easy to bring the penis into contact with it from a variety of positions throughout the course of lovemaking.

Although knowing the exact location of the Grafenberg Spot will not make or break a relationship, it will definitely enhance your sexual pleasure. Listen to what Thomas R. related to me about his experience with the Grafenberg Spot.

"Diana and I had been dating each other for about six or seven months, and we both regarded our sexual relationship as quite good. She regularly had one or two orgasms whenever we made love—which was about three or four times a week. They were mainly clitoral orgasms, but occasionally a vaginal orgasm as well.

"Then Diana read an article about the Grafenberg Spot that told how to locate the spot inside the vagina. When she was able to conclusively locate the spot on her own, she

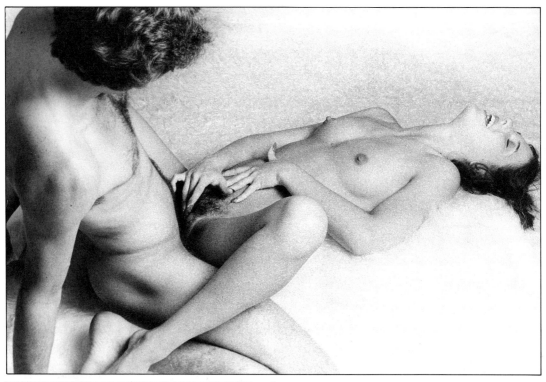

position was one where Diana was on her knees, her sexy ass tilted up toward me, her legs spread so that they were just a little more than shoulder width apart. When I placed a hand on each hip, just below her waist, I was able to control the movement. As I thrust in and out of her, and as she moved undulatingly, she would tell me when the tip of my penis was in contact with the Grafenberg Spot. Interestingly, unlike what some people would think, it is not necessarily at the point of deepest penetration. Naturally, this depends on the physical structure of both partners' anatomy.

"Every time I hit the 'spot,' she would moan and shudder. That night Diana had more orgasms than she had ever experienced before, and she said she felt as though she were 'tingling all over.'

"The benefits from Diana's point of view are obvious, but I derived benefit from it as well. Seeing my lover in such ecstacy is a real turn-on. Also, the knowledge that I can thoroughly and predictably please my lover so well has bolstered my confidence, not only in my relationship with Diana but in my overall self-image."

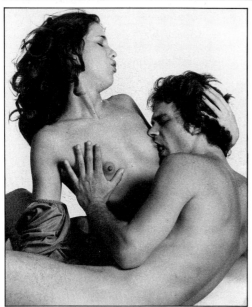

shared her revelation with me and showed me how to locate it as well with my finger.

"That night in bed we experimented with different positions that 'hit the spot.' Our favorite

VISIONS OF LOVE

Assume, for the moment, the role of a voyeur. Close your eyes and travel back into your thoughts to that first moment of innocence when the curve of a buttock or the hardness of a nipple aroused you to a level of flushed excitement. We are overwhelmed, in our day-to-day existence, with the politics and etiquette of sexual expression. This chapter is devoted to the primal response in every human being, to the beauty and power of two people making love. Observe the magic of intimacy and arousal with the rich passion of vision as only a photographer who reaches for the truth of expression can record. Be in love with love itself, and allow these erotic images to arouse and transport you.

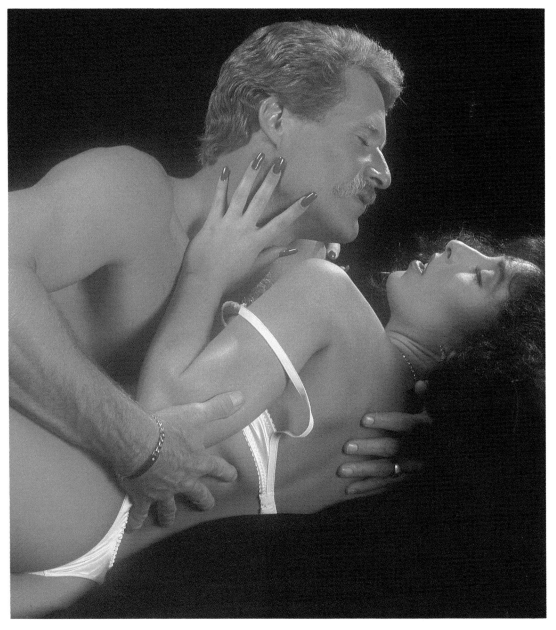

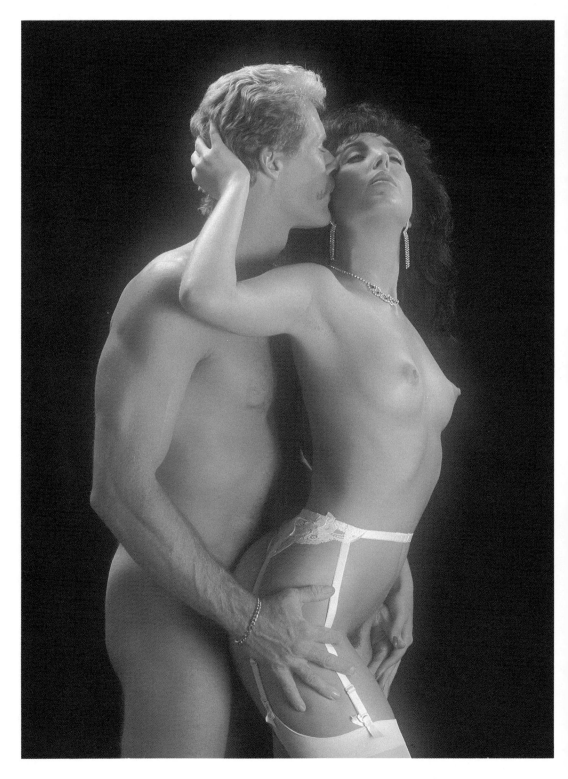

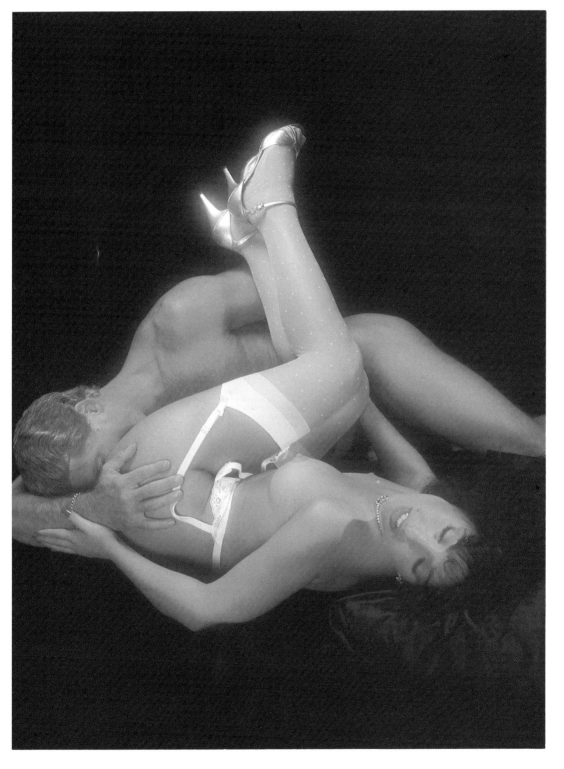

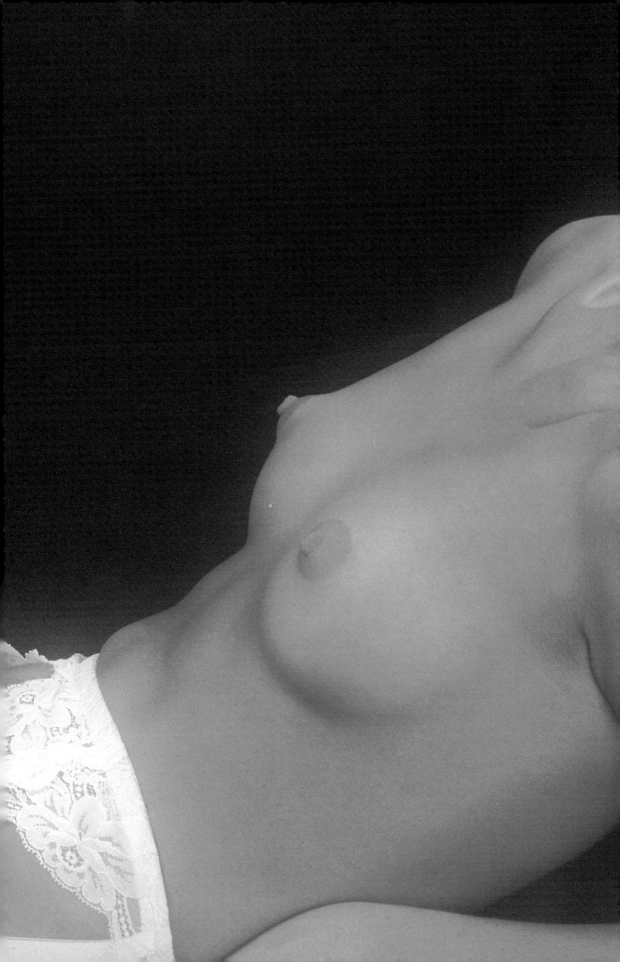

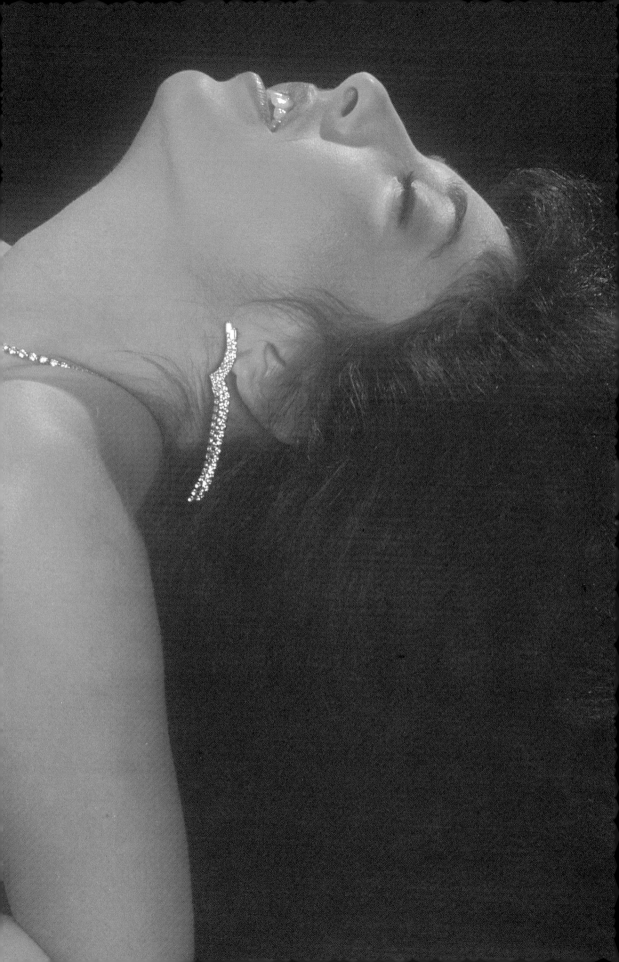

VISIONS

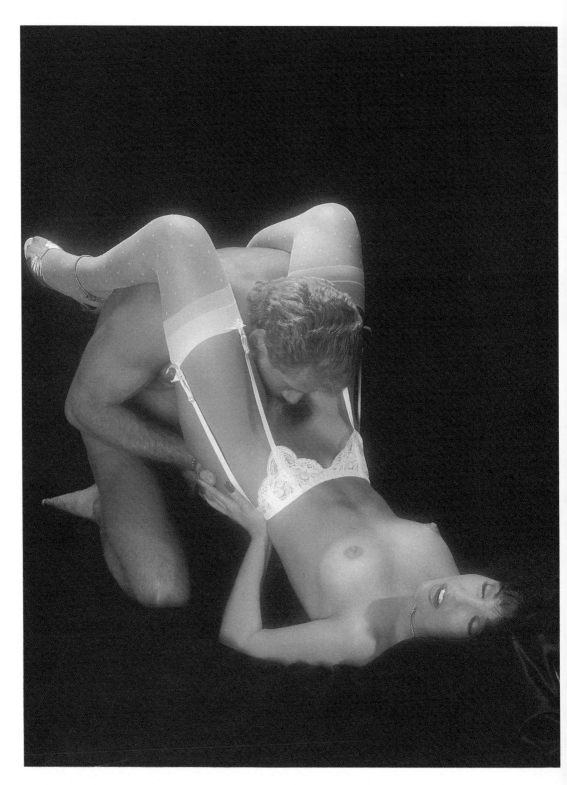

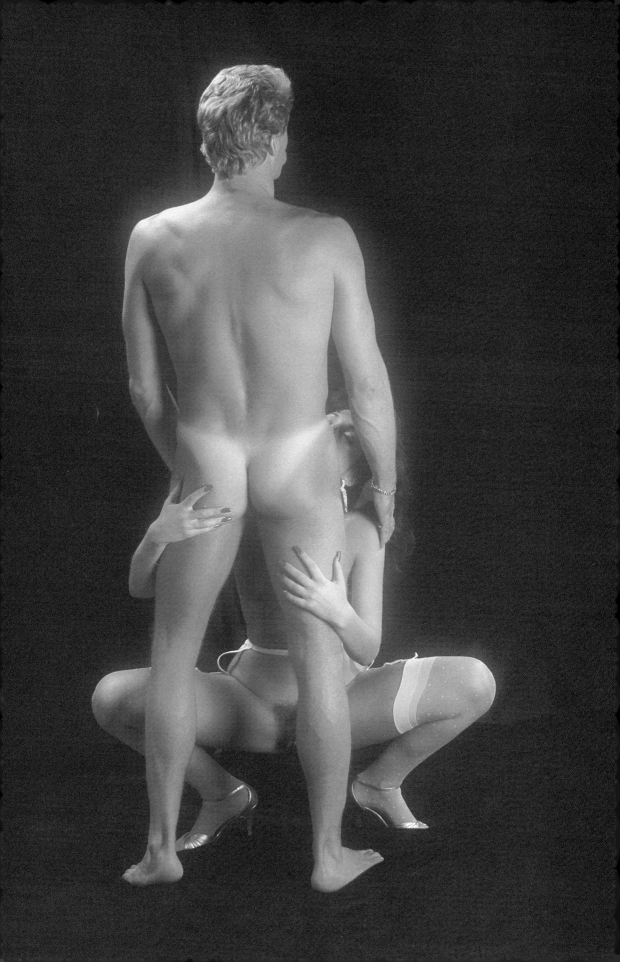

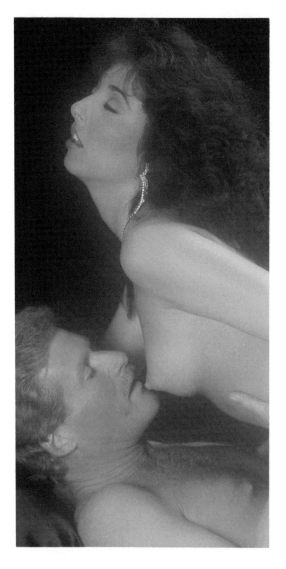
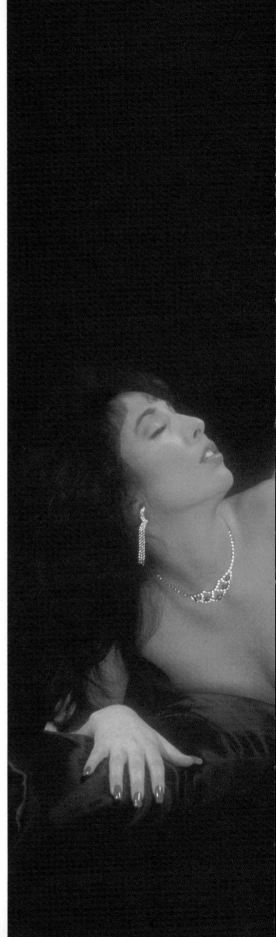

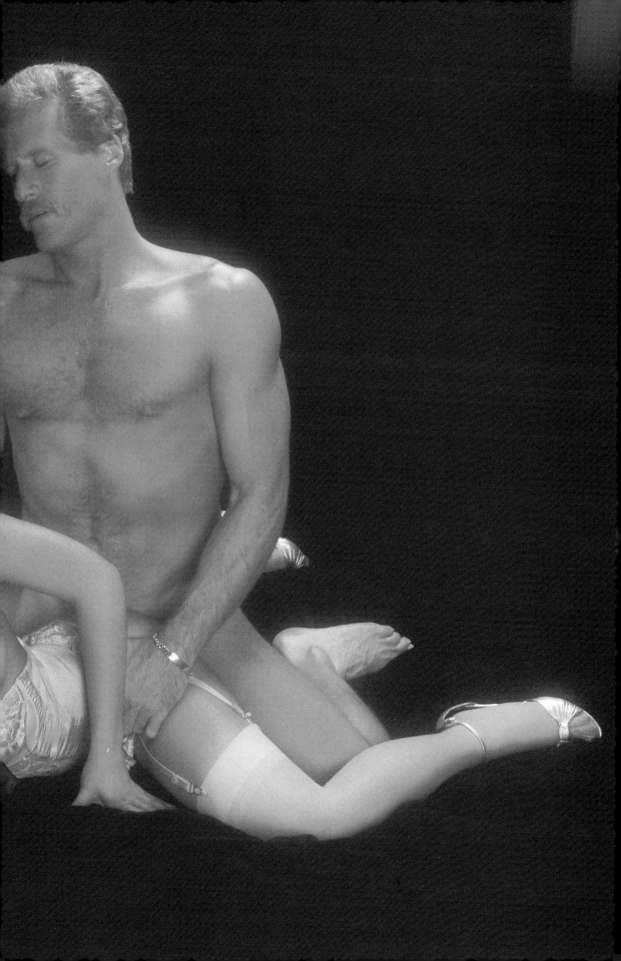

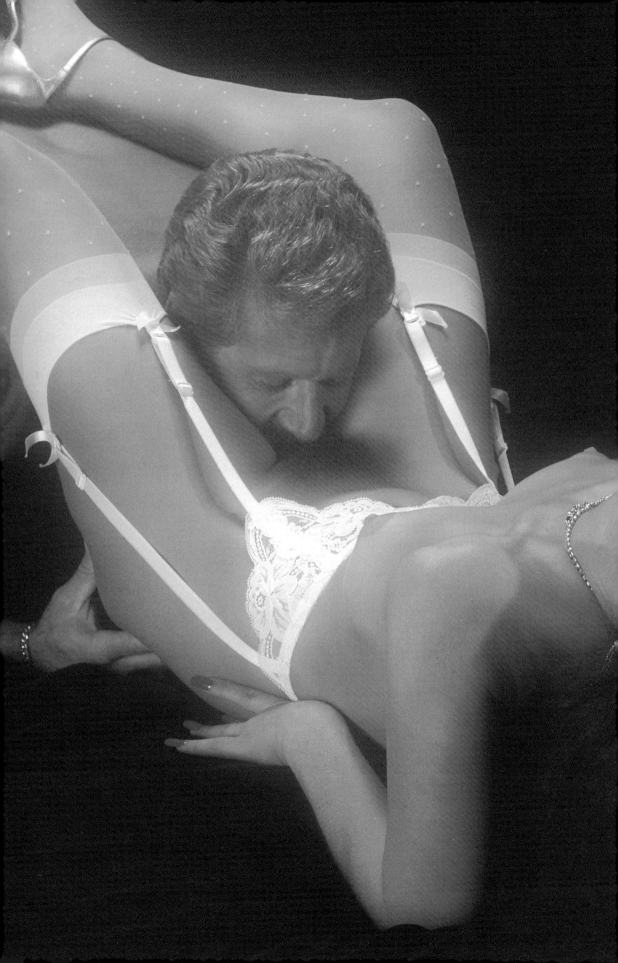

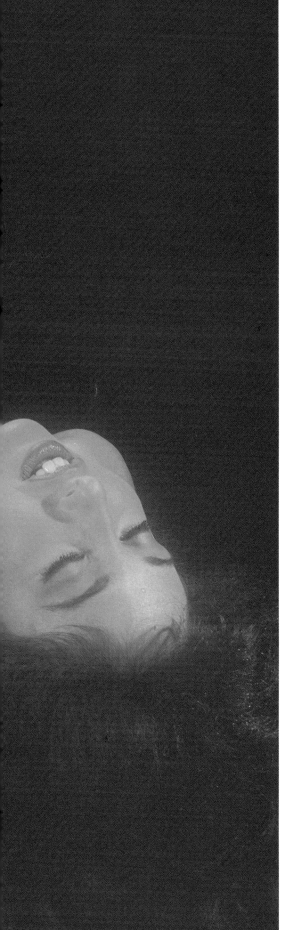

VISIONS

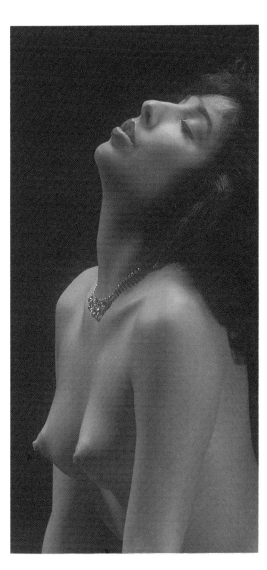

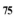

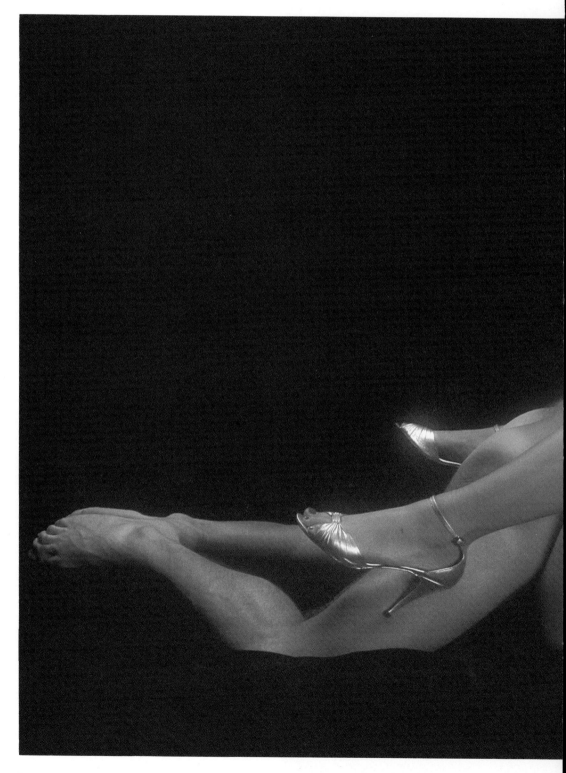

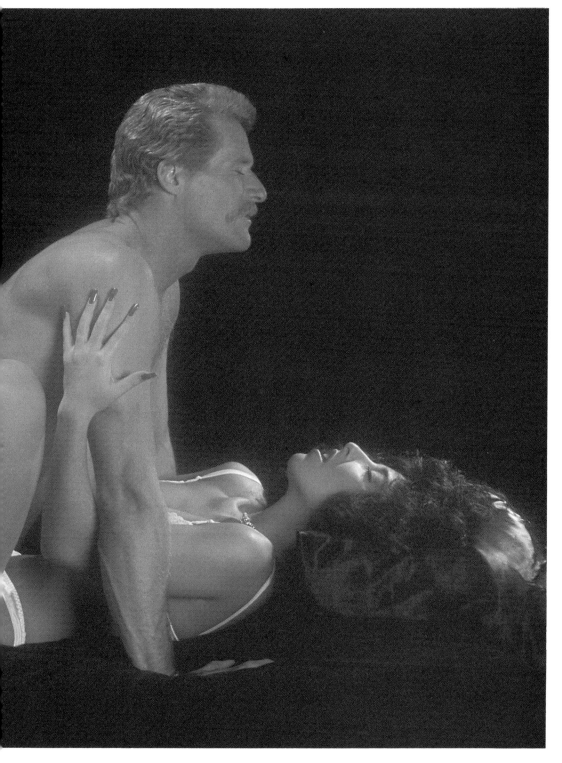

VISIONS

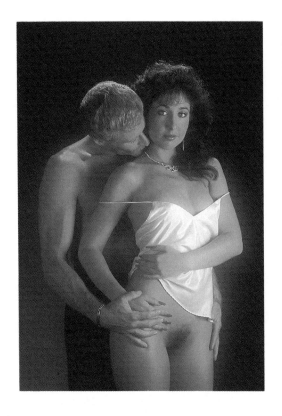

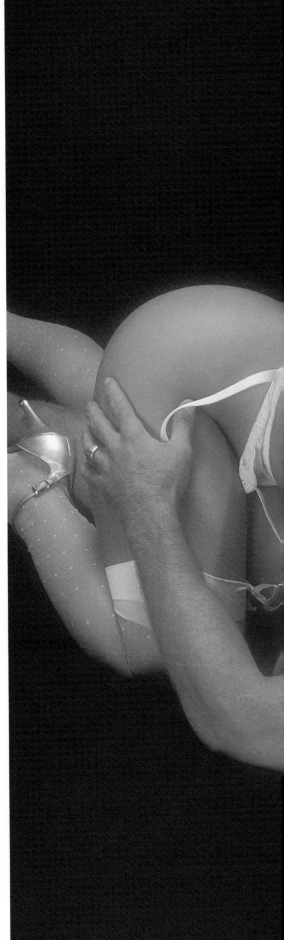

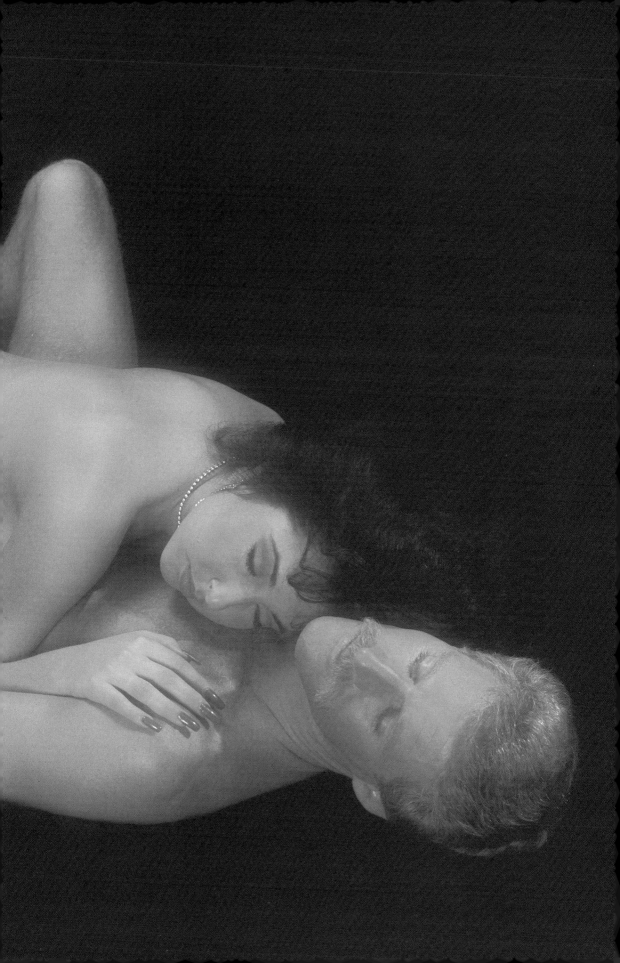

VISIONS

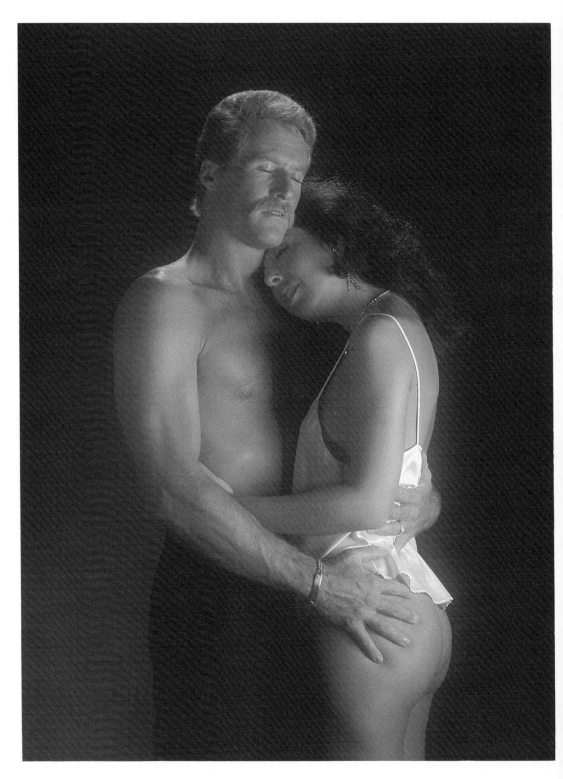

BASIC·SEXUAL·POSITIONS

MAN ON TOP

Long ago and far away, there lived an unmarried woman by the name of Agnes Shunnary, a beautiful young woman whose red hair and green eyes would have qualified her for Irish citizenship had there been an Ireland at that time. But alas, there was no such country way back then.

People thought very differently about things than we do now. For example, clothes were merely for protection, and during the warm summer months, people often eschewed clothes altogether. Another aspect of their society worthy of note was that sex was often performed in public.

One afternoon while sitting around the park watching an afternoon's live-sex activity, the attendant crowd was treated to an event that would have earth-shattering consequences. Young Agnes, so proud of her supple young body, was about to perform sex with her partner when she was struck with a brilliant idea. Until this time, sex had always—always—been performed with the woman on her knees and the man entering her from behind. After all, the people said, this is how the animals do it. But then, the animals often peed on trees, which the people almost never did. They were well on their way to becoming civilized.

On this afternoon, as Agnes's partner approached her, she stunned the assembled multitude—and especially her partner—by turning over, lying flat on her back, and spreading her legs. At first her stunned partner was confused by the change in script and initially tried to sit on her. However, Agnes had apparently figured the whole thing out in advance and quickly guided her partner to the safety of her sexual orifice.

Although the crowd was initially silent, they finally erupted with appreciative applause. In fact, what Agnes initiated that day became popular throughout the land almost immediately.

To show their gratitude, the people actually named this new position after Miss Shunnary. It has carried on to this day and is known, after a slight translation, as the Missionary Position.

As I've said before, it's not always easy separating fact from fiction when it comes to sex. Regardless of its derivation, the most common sexual position is the missionary position, or the

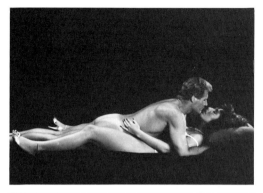

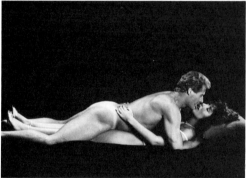

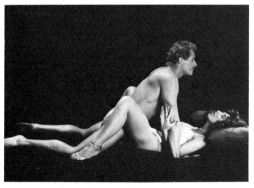

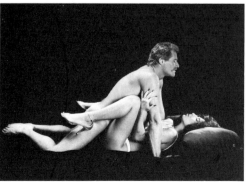

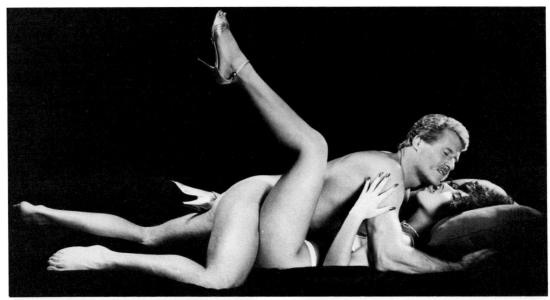

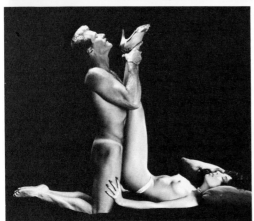

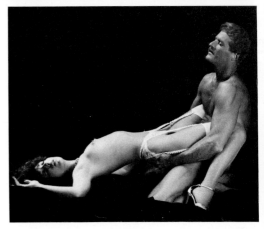

man-on-top, no-frills position. This position has taken a lot of heat in the recent past and is harangued almost as often as Burbank in Johnny Carson monologues.

This basic position allows direct clitoral stimulation by the penis shaft and/or pubic bone. It allows lovers to look into each other's eyes and to kiss each other on the mouth. It also enable the woman to control, to a certain extent, the degree of penetration by the man's penis. This can be done by either hollowing the back or curving it up toward her partner. Hollowing the back limits how far in the penis can go, while lifting and curving the pelvis up toward the penis allows for deeper penetration.

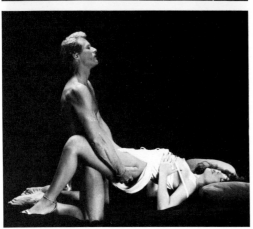

By simply moving her legs into various arrangements from this basic position, the woman can greatly enhance her partner's pleasure as well as her own. For example, if she closes her legs tightly once her lover's penis is inside her, the woman will substantially increase the amount of friction and, therefore, sensation on her labia and clitoris. This position also creates greater pressure on the penis, thereby strengthening the man's erection. This position is good for a man with a long and narrow penis, as well as a woman with a wide vagina.

Just by moving the legs, or rearranging them, all kinds of different depths and sensations can be produced. For example, with the woman's legs spread apart, the man can pull himself deeply into his lover. Again with the man on top, from a position where both his legs are within his lover's spread legs, if the man lifts his left leg to allow his lover's right leg to move

between his legs, a wide range of leverage and depth can be achieved. This position makes it easy to stimulate the clitoris—so much so, in fact, that both partners would be wise to monitor their lovemaking activities in this position because both can get rubbed raw by the intense friction that may be generated.

A woman can also spread her legs wider apart and even put one or both of her legs over her lover's shoulders. The most common position of this type is with the woman's legs spread slightly, bent at the knee so that the soles of her feet lie flat on the bed. This allows fairly deep penile penetration, while the vulva is stimulated at the same time.

Another common variation of the same position is with the woman's legs raised, feet off the bed, knees and thighs tilted back toward her chest. This position allows for even deeper penetration and is, therefore, particularly good for

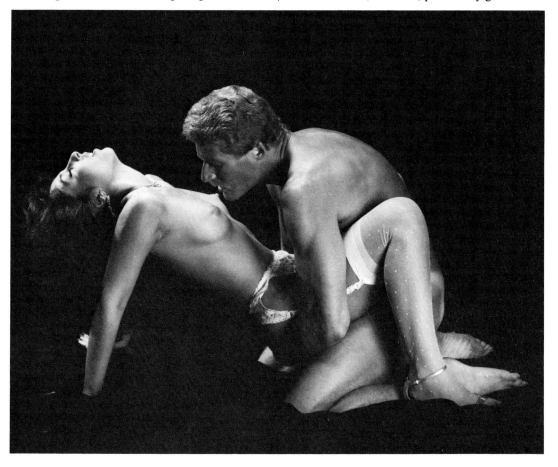

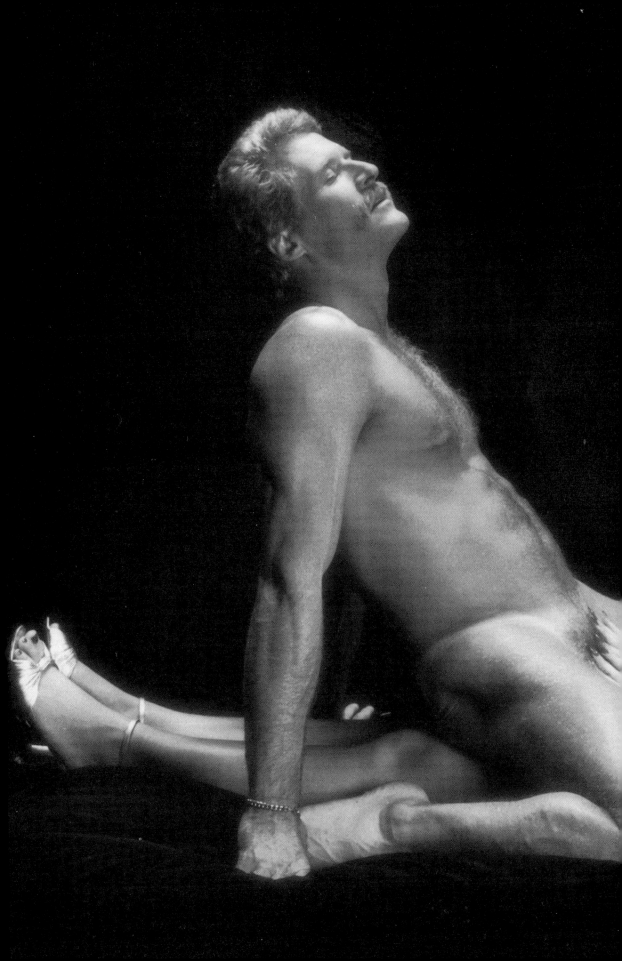

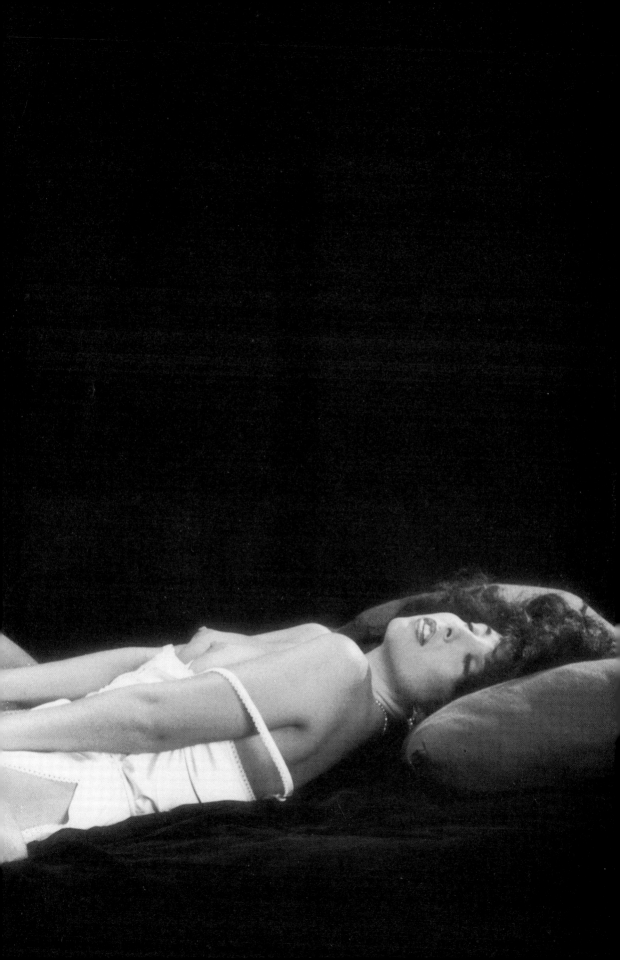

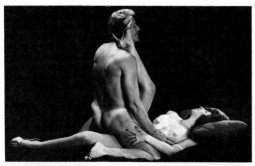

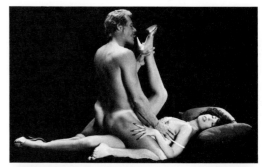

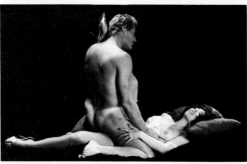

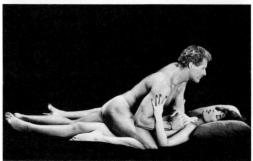

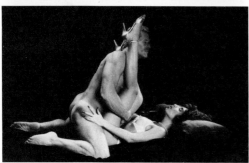

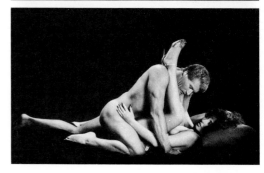

men with smaller penises. Don't be ashamed to use this position just because of that, though. It's also a good position for men with average-size penises. It is not, however, an ideal position for a man with a large penis and a woman with a small vagina.

Other variations involve placement of the woman's legs. She can lift them and put them over her lover's shoulders. She can wrap her legs around her lover's waist, crossing them at the ankles. These positions have things in common. They allow for deep penetration. And, except for the position where the woman crosses her ankles, they put the woman in control. With her legs, she can keep the man from penetrating too deeply, or she can relax her legs and to allow him to go as deeply as possible.

The man may wish to cup his lover's buttocks, while her legs are over his shoulders or sticking straight up at a right angle to her torso, and lift. This gives control of the depth of penetration back to the man.

Another variation of the man-on-top position begins with the woman lying flat on her back and the man on his knees between her legs. He then turns the woman on her side, so that her bottom leg runs underneath him and between his legs, while her upper leg is either over his shoulder or bent and dangling over one of his thighs. Although this comes close to a rear-entry position, it is not. By holding his lover's lower buttock with one hand and her opposite hip with the other, the man is able to manipulate the rhythm and depth of insertion. It also

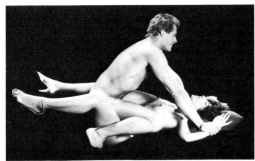

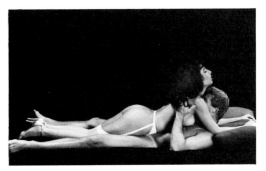

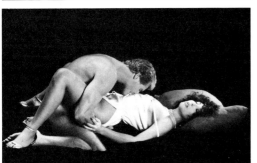

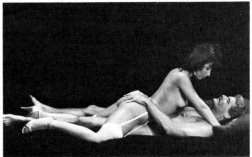

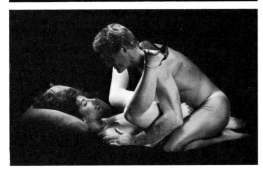

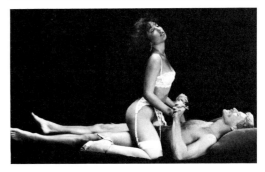

gives him a wonderful bird's-eye view of his lover in profile—her legs, abdomen, and breasts. At his option, the man may choose to raise the upper leg, which not only allows him greater penetration, but also provides an excellent view of his penis being swallowed by his lover's vulva. Certain positions lend themselves better than others to being able to see the sex organs in action. Personally, I find this quite stimulating.

Another man-on-top position that affords the man a great view of the action is one where he kneels between his lover's legs. After inserting his penis, he then lifts the woman's hips off the bed up "onto" his erection.

WOMAN ON TOP
Positions that call for the woman to be on top

not only provide a nice change of pace, they also are quite practical for a number of reasons. First, such positions turn control back over to the woman, who can often guide herself to orgasm by positioning herself and the penis in the most stimulating positions. Second, the man is now free to fondle his lover's breasts and clitoris.

The most common of these positions calls for the man to lie flat on his back while the woman kneels and straddles his penis, her knees on either side of the man's hips. Thomas B. explains why this is one of his favorite positions.

"I'd been dating Joanne for only a few weeks, and our sex, though fairly uninventive, was pretty good. One night Joanne told me she wanted to try something a little different from

the basic positions we'd been using. So she got on top of me, straddled my penis, curling her knees underneath her. We'd been making love for about a half hour before she got on top of me. When she did, the love sweat dripping down her face, chest and breasts glistened in the candlelight, it was quite a turn-on.

"Then she uncurled her legs, stretching her legs out straight so that her feet wound up at about my shoulders. The position made the muscles in her thighs tighten up and her legs looked absolutely fantastic. I propped my head up with a pillow to take it all in. Besides her fabulous-looking legs and her breasts, I could also see my penis sticking up and disappearing into Joanne's pretty little pussy.

"I reached out and grabbed her underneath her knees with each hand and began to alternately pull her toward me, then push her away. The sensation of that plus the sight of all of Joanne's femininity all at once was just too much for me, and I had one of the best orgasms of my life.

"We've incorporated that position into our regular sexual routine. And sometimes, when I get to taking Joanne a little too much for granted, all I have to do is see her from that perspective and I remember what a great-looking woman she really is."

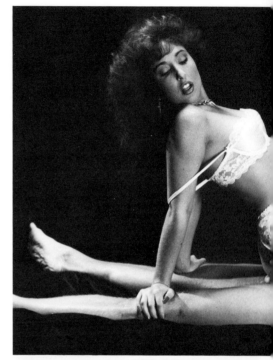

With the woman on top, straddling her lover, legs curled underneath her, she can control the focus of stimulation by leaning forward or bending backward. If she leans forward, the clitoris receives more stimulation. If she leans backward, vaginal stimulation is increased.

Another variation on this basic position is to have the woman turn around and face away from her lover. This position, with the woman's anus toward the man's face, can be visually stimulating to the male. As the female bends forward toward the man's toes, her vulva, which is full of the man's penis, and her anus are totally—and I mean totally—exposed to her partner. But even more important than that, considerable pressure is brought to bear on the penis from this position.

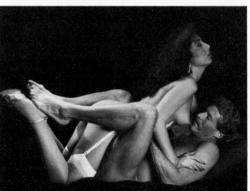

A variation on this from-behind straddling position is for the woman to uncurl her legs and stretch them back so that her lover can, by cupping her thighs from underneath, control the action.

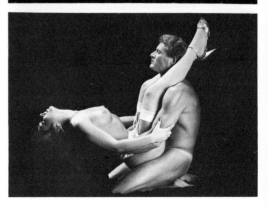

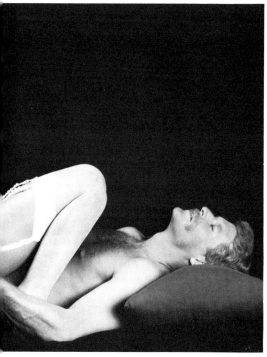

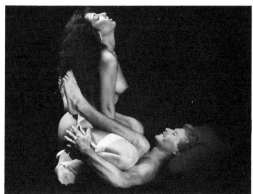

SIDE BY SIDE

Side-by-side positions can be very intimate. For the most part, these positions—except in some of their most acrobatic variations—are for people who like to cuddle. Spooning may be a term familiar to you. What it means is to cuddle up with someone, both of you lying on your side facing the same direction, with one body wrapped around the other, so that one person's lap becomes like a spoon cradling the other person's bottom. With the man in back, cuddling in this position can easily lead to intercourse.

This position can also provide unexpected

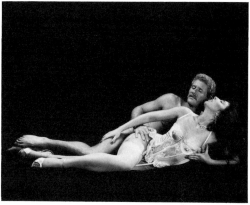

benefits, as shown in the story of Allan H.

"When I first started dating after my wife and I got divorced, it was a case of willing spirit and weak flesh. I was interested in women—very interested—but I just wasn't used to the dating scene and the pressure that goes with it, in terms of bedroom performance.

"I didn't find it difficult to get dates; I'm a good-looking guy. And all the time my wife and I were together—almost ten years—I never had a problem 'getting it up.' My big problem after my divorce was confidence. I'd lost a great deal of it when my marriage failed. My wife was the only woman I'd ever been with. What it boiled down to was that I knew I could do it with my wife, but I wasn't sure about anybody else.

"My first experience was a horrible one. I went out with a girl from work and we ended up in bed, but I couldn't get it up. She said she understood, but I could tell she was disappointed. I was too embarrassed even to ask her out again.

"The next date I had, the same thing happened. By the morning after my second date, I was ready to swear off women. I was just too scared.

"Then I met Raegina. I really liked her. Not only was I attracted to her, but we hit it off in every way possible. We laughed a lot together, liked the same movies, music, everything.

"When it came time to hit the sack—and I tried to put it off as long as I could—I was scared to death. I didn't want to blow it. Unfortunately, the pressure of really wanting it to work with Raegina was just too much. We went to bed, and the same thing happened—or, more precisely, didn't happen. She was very under-

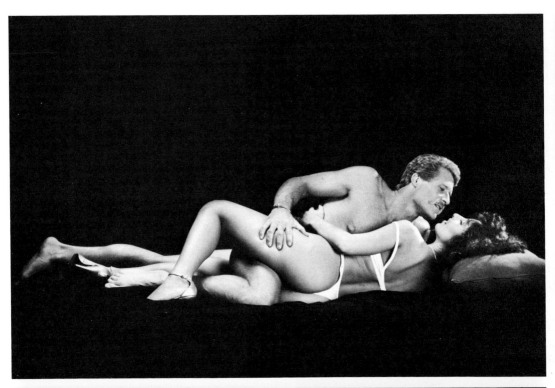

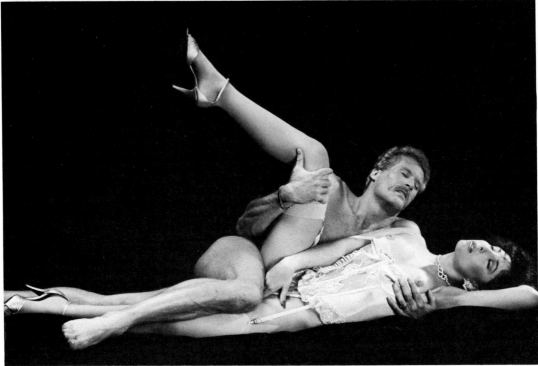

standing, but I was devastated.

"About an hour later, I was lying there wide awake, my mind spinning. I just couldn't sleep. Raegina was asleep, and I was cuddled up behind her as she lay on her side. I looked at her as she slept, and she looked so beautiful. And all of a sudden, guess what? I started to get hard, and from the position I was in, my penis almost crawled up inside her without even having to move. It was the start of something fantastic. Since that night, I haven't had any problems whatsoever in the sex department.

"I thought about everything the next morning, and I realized what had happened. First, I had no pressure to perform; Raegina was already asleep. Second, she was lying in a position where I didn't have to wake her up to get things going. If I'd had to wake her up, the pressure probably would have started all over again. But since she was lying there on her side, her sexy little buns sticking out, her sweet pussy exposed to me, it was a perfect opportunity for me to get hard and get inside her without the pressure of having to perform."

One little addendum to Allan's story: if your partner's vagina is not already lubricated, it can be a rude awakening to just jam your penis inside it while she's sleeping. If she's not moist and ready, use some lubricant on your penis. You'll find your partner will be much more receptive.

Many women, and men, enjoy being awakened by their partner with the sex act already— or partially—underway. It can be dreamy and fun. And it beats the hell out of an alarm clock.

X MARKS THE SPOT

Another group of positions that can be fun to experiment with start with the basic position as follows. The woman lies flat on her back and lifts her legs. The man lies on his side, facing the woman at an angle perpendicular to her so that their bodies cross in the middle. The woman's feet come to rest on the man's hip or thigh. From this position, the man then enters her.

This position offers several advantages. First, the man does not have to support his weight. Second, there is the exciting feeling that, if the woman draws her knees into her chest rather than resting her feet on her partner's hip or

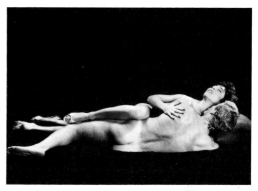

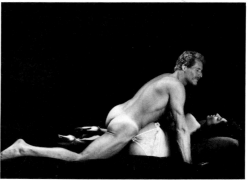

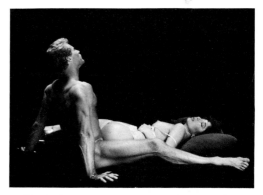

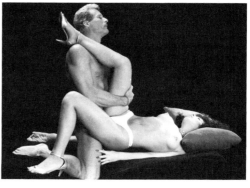

thighs, the only point at which the couple is joined is at the genitals.

Many couples find this an exquisite position in which to achieve orgasm. Because the two partners are joined only at the genitals, the genitals become the focus of sensation. Another advantage of this position is that both of the woman's hands are free to caress her own breasts or stimulate her clitoris in order to help bring herself to orgasm. One—and sometimes both—of the man's hands are also free to do these things or anything else he may choose to do to give his lover pleasure.

A variation of this position is for the man, from the same basic position, to spread his lover's farthest leg out as far as it will go, while at the same time wrapping her other leg around his shoulder. This still leaves the woman with both hands free, while giving both partners an exhilaratingly explicit view of each other's genitals.

THE RHYTHM OF LOVE

And now, a word about rhythm. Many of you already realize that music wasn't meant just to be danced to. Rock and roll, rhythm and blues, and many other kinds of music can provide an excellent backdrop for lovemaking.

The beat that works best for you and your lover will be something you work out through experience. Some men and women enjoy deep, constant thrusts done to a double-time beat, while others enjoy slow, shallow thrusts. The best gauge of the love tempo for you and your lover is your own response.

Experiment, read erotic literature, and learn what others say about interesting ways to make love. You've got nothing to lose. Most of us are willing to educate ourselves about such things as computers, baseball players' averages, and stock market quotes. Yet none of these things can really play as satisfying a part in our daily lives as a happy and enjoyable sex life with someone we love.

As you look through this book and others, you may find some positions that look better than others to you. Just because one book claims to describe *the* position to end all positions should not make any difference to you. The only thing that should matter is how it feels to you and your lover.

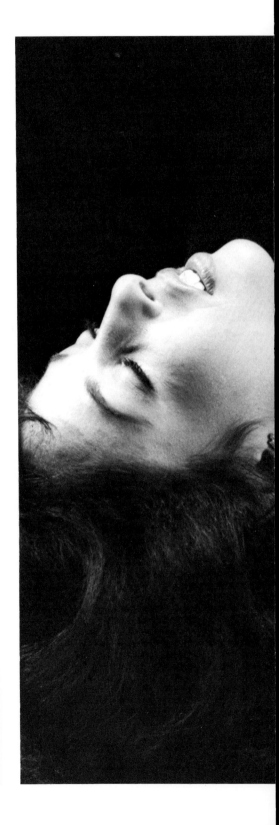

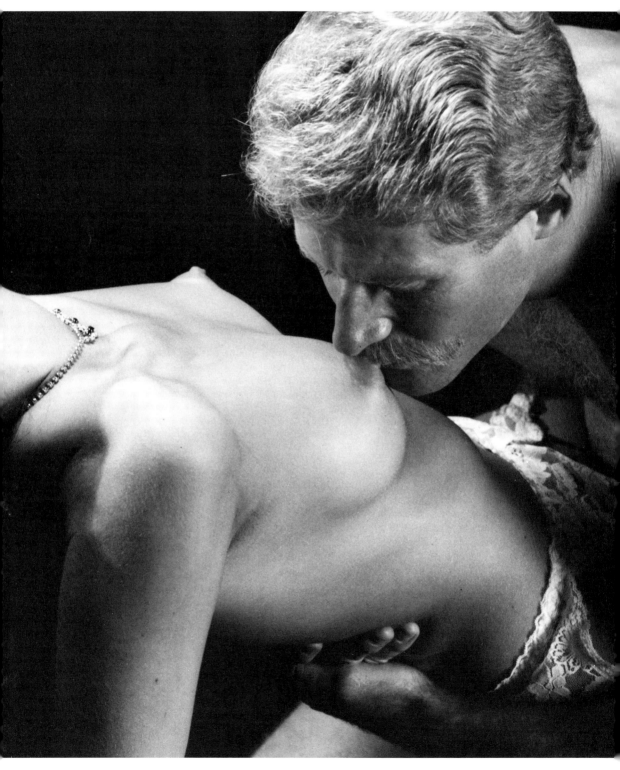

REAR-ENTRY·POSITIONS

Even though the missionary position has remained the most popular position in which to make love, the rear-entry position is currently enjoying a surge in popularity. But then, the rear-entry position was probably the original number-one position long ago. After all, when's the last time you saw a couple of dogs in the missionary position?

A major appeal of the rear-entry position is its visual dynamics for the male. The woman is vulnerable and subservient in stance: leaning forward, head on the floor or pillow, resting on her elbows, exposing her sex organs and her anus to her lover, who, with both hands firmly on each of his lover's hips, is totally in control of the action.

This position is also the best in which to conceive. A word of caution, however: men with longer penises must be careful not to hurt their partners because penetration can reach its maximum in certain variations of this position.

Most women enjoy this position as much as men. Whether or not the woman feels vulnerable or subservient—which she may or may not enjoy—penetration is deep in this position, and chances of hitting the Grafenberg Spot are greatly increased over front-facing positions.

Tim R. has another reason why he particularly likes this position.

"My girlfriend, Penny, has a great ass. I mean, it's the kind of ass that, in a pair of short shorts—which she just about lives in during the summer—can cause a lot of tires to squeal. The first time I ever saw her, I visualized what it would be like to do it to her from behind. Those were great fantasies, but they were nothing compared to what it was like when I really got to make love with her.

"When she gets on her knees and I get inside her from behind, I'm in heaven. Even after we've made love for a while and I'm tired, all I have to do is roll her over, get inside her, look at her ass, and I'm rock-hard again. I spread her beautiful cheeks apart and look at her cute little asshole. Sometimes I smack her on her ass—not too hard, just enough to get a response out of her, which is usually a low moan.

"Penny loves getting it from behind as much as I like giving it to her. She likes to take my cock deep inside her. And I think she likes flaunting her little ass up in the air the way

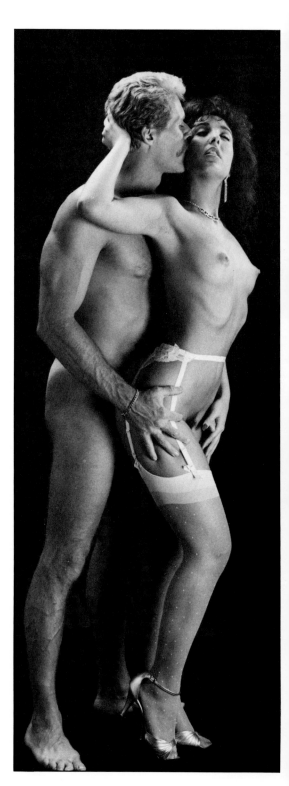

*she does when I'm just about ready to get
inside her.*

"It's definitely our favorite position."

Variations of this position—woman on her
knees, man inside her from behind—involve
playing around with different leg arrangements.
For example, instead of having the woman's
legs between her lover's, she can move them to
the outside, as her lover closes his legs together.
In a slight variation of this position, the woman
can extend one leg out behind her while sliding
the other knee up toward her shoulder.

Another advantage of these positions is
that the man can reach around and under
his partner to cup and caress her breasts.
Because the action is often fast and furious in
this position, and because the breasts are totally
unencumbered, they often swing freely, thus
providing another exciting visual image for the
man, who can simply tilt his head to the right
or left to watch the breasts in motion.

NON-KNEELING REAR-ENTRY POSITIONS

A woman flat on her stomach with her legs
spread apart is an extremely provocative invita-
tion to almost any man. As with all positions,
this one has its advantages and disadvantages.
One disadvantage is that unless the woman is
extremely conscious of tilting her pelvis in the
right direction, the man cannot penetrate very
deeply and can, in fact, become easily dis-
lodged. There are several ways to remedy this.
The most common is to put a pillow under the
woman's lower abdomen, thereby providing the
tilt needed for easy and deep penetration.

In sex, as in real-estate speculation, leverage
is everything. Michael W. seems to understand
this as well as anyone.

*"I enjoyed having sex with my girlfriend from
behind. The problem was, I never could get
enough leverage to sustain an erection for any
period of time. This was a very frustrating situation. What made it doubly trying was the fact
that Nancy, my girlfriend, found it easier to
have an orgasm getting it from behind than
any other way.*

*"One afternoon while we were making love, I
was inside Nancy from behind and we were very
near the right edge of the bed. I started to lose
my balance, my right leg went off the bed, and*

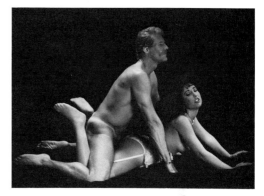

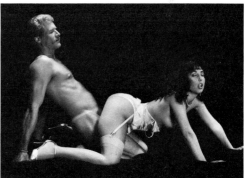

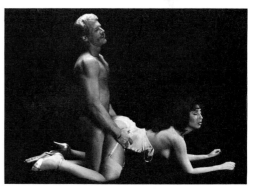

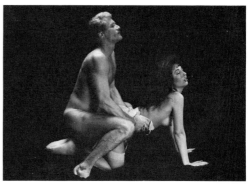

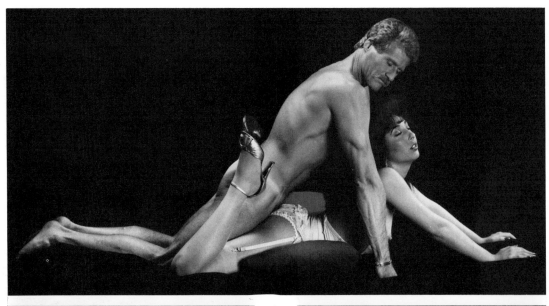

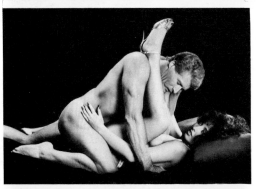

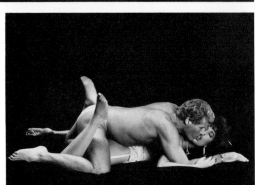

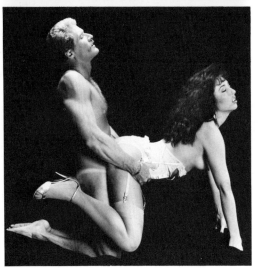

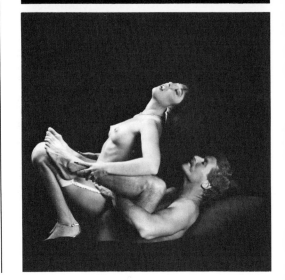

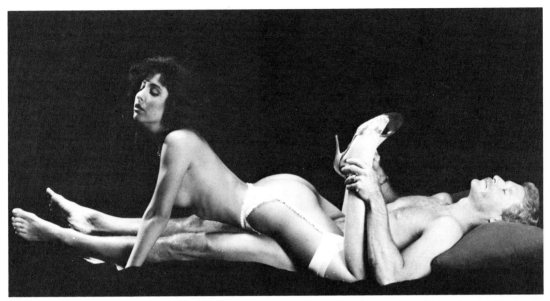

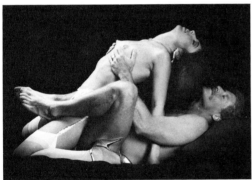

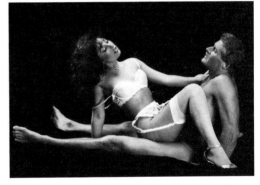

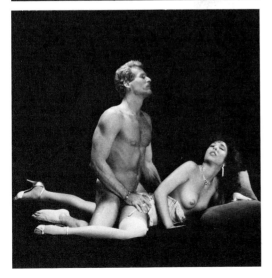

my foot landed flat on the floor. An amazing thing happened as I tried to re-situate myself. I found that by playing around with how I positioned my right foot, I could gain considerable leverage with my penis. We made love for about forty-five minutes in that position, and Nancy came like crazy several times.

"Since then, that position has become one of our favorites."

Speaking of leverage, there are several female-superior, rear-entry positions that, with the proper amount of leverage, can be quite satisfying. For example, with the man lying on his back, legs spread, the woman, with her back to her partner, can "sit down" on his penis. In this position, it is easy to adjust the degree of leverage and penetration to maximize the enjoyment of both parties.

A GENTLEMAN ALWAYS OFFERS HIS SEAT TO A LADY

In this position, the man kneels on the bed, sitting on his heels, penis erect. Then he guides his lover, who has her back to him, to her seat—which is on his penis. This position can also accommodate the woman facing her lover, if she simply wraps her legs around him as she takes his penis inside her.

STAND BY YOUR MAN

Another excellent rear-entry position is with both partners standing. Women who are shorter than their lovers may need to wear high-heeled shoes to compensate for the difference in height. Don't worry, if you want to make love in this position, you can work it out. Larry G. will testify to that.

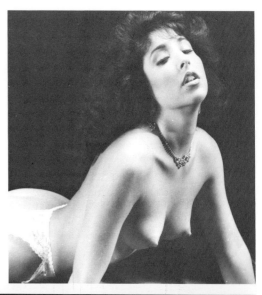

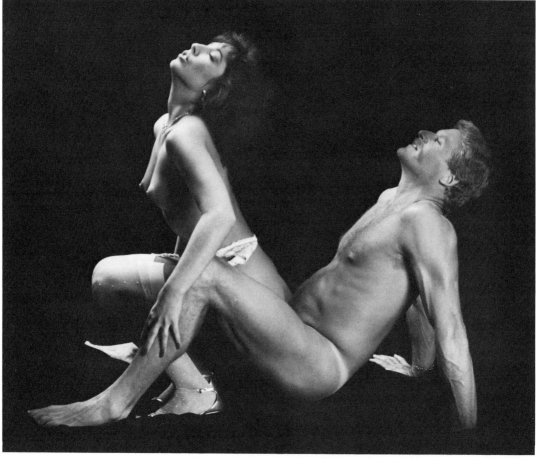

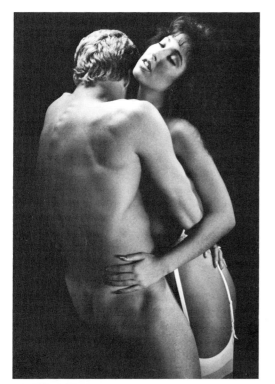

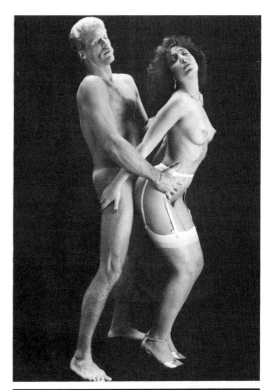

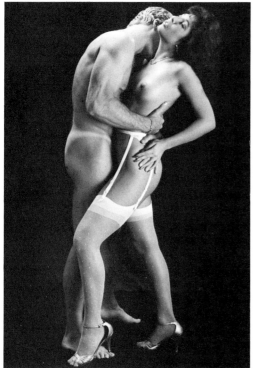

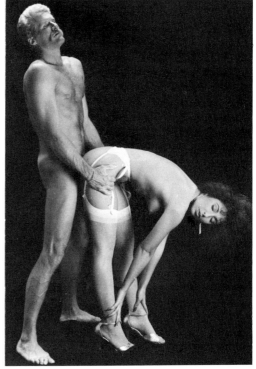

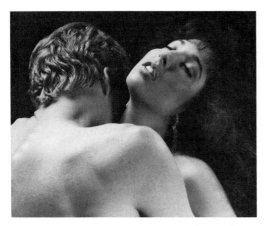

"My girlfriend, Rita, works out a lot at the local health club, and she's in great shape. In fact, she even teaches classes there sometimes.

"She's got a key to my place, and she sometimes gets home before I do. One night I was working late at the office and didn't get home until about nine. When I opened the door, I saw Rita standing in the kitchen putting the last touches on a crab salad. But what really got my attention was the way she was dressed. She was wearing high-heeled shoes and her black leotard. Let me tell you about this leotard. First of all, it's got little more than a string in back that goes up the crack in Rita's ass. Second, instead of a full top in front, it's got thin straps that start about stomach level and go over the shoulders. Obviously, a shirt is supposed to be worn underneath. But Rita wasn't wearing anything except the shoes and the leotard. She looked at me and asked if I was hungry. I was hungry all right, but not for food.

"I took her hand and led her into the living room, watching the way her body moved in those high-heeled shoes. The lights were already dimmed to accentuate the mood. She undressed me and gave me head. Then we did something we'd never done before. We'd often had sex with me entering her from behind, but always while she was kneeling or lying on her stomach. Tonight she took my hand and led me to one of the dining room chairs. She leaned over the chair, stuck her ass up in the air, and spread her cheeks with her hands. I slid aside the string that ran up the crack in her ass and stuck my cock into her vagina. With a hand on each of her cheeks, I felt totally in control of her body.

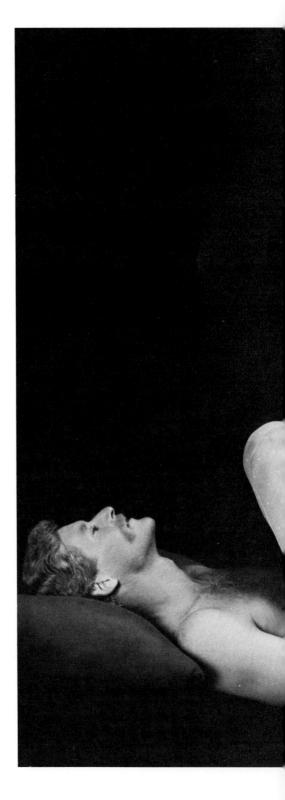

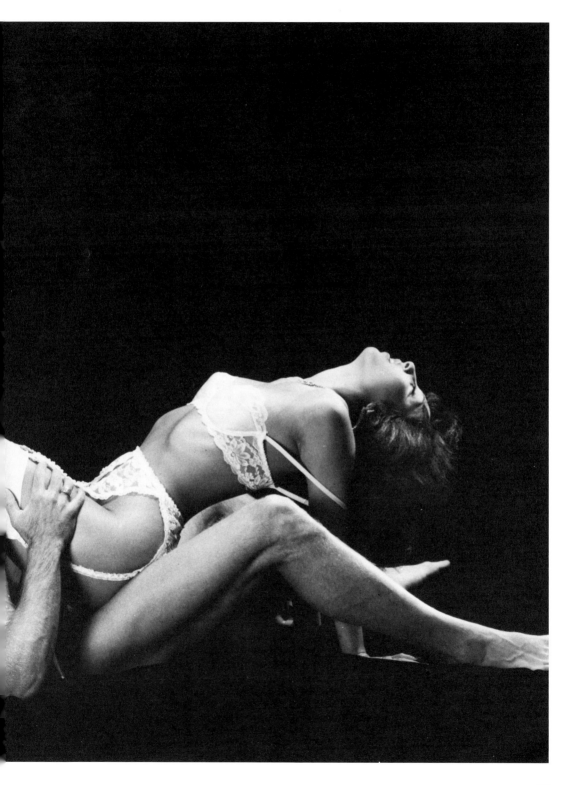

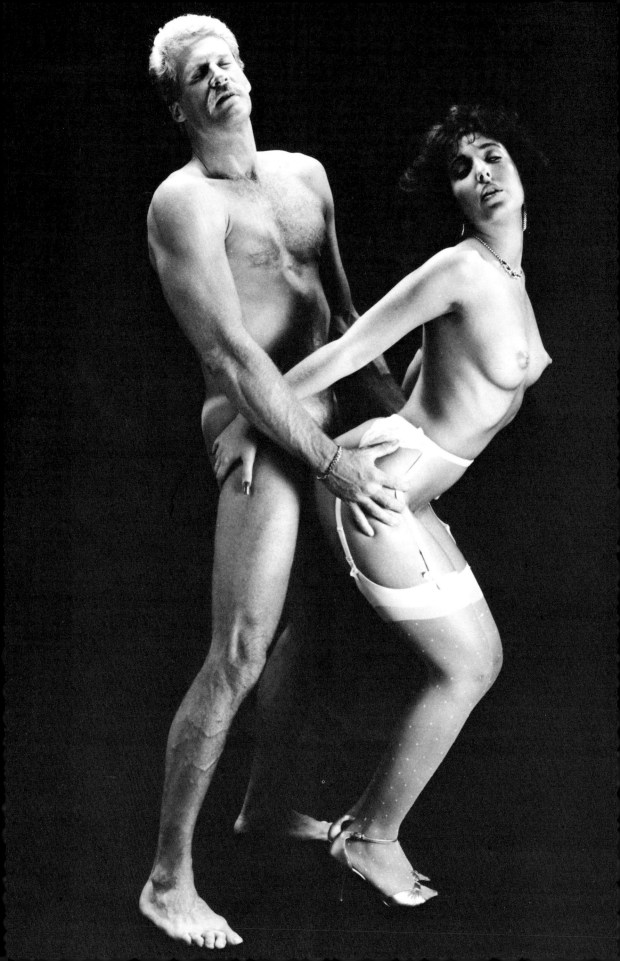

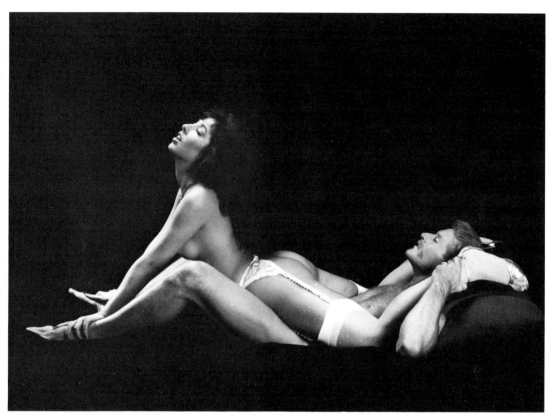

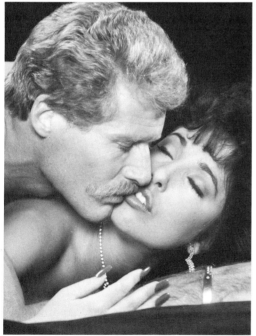

"Looking down on Rita's fabulous, tanned legs, lightly muscled and shaped because she was still wearing her high-heeled shoes, I got an incredible rush. I'd always loved her ass and legs, but I'd never seen them from exactly this perspective—looking down on them while I was pumping away inside her.

"After a while, she moved away from the chair and bent down even further, so that her nose was touching her knees and her hands were actually grasping the backs of my knees— as I said, Rita's in great shape. Meanwhile, her pussy was tilted almost straight up, my cock throbbing with excitement, still pumping away inside it. I could hardly believe my eyes. Rita looked incredible!"

ANAL SEX

Despite its lack of wide acceptance, anal sex actually has several things to recommend it as a sexual change of pace. First, the anus is almost always a "tighter fit" than the vagina, thus providing the man with increased friction anytime

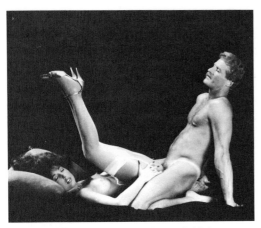

he enters his partner anally. Second, if the man has his penis in his partner's vagina and his finger, or fingers, in her anus, he can massage one with the other through the pelvic floor, which is a pocket of sensation for his partner.

Many men mention that since anal sex is still considered taboo in a society that is quickly running out of such things, anal sex provides a special thrill.

If you're going to try anal sex, there are a few things to keep in mind. First and foremost, remember that, because of the opposite chemical nature of the rectum and vagina, **anything (penis, finger, vibrator) that is inserted into the rectum must be carefully washed before it is inserted into the vagina to avoid infection.**

Another very important thing to remember is lubrication. Even if a woman is willing, the moment can be ruined because, without proper lubrication, the entire process is simply too painful.

The keys to successful anal sex, especially the first time, are mental preparation and taking it slowly. Consider the experience of John R.

"I'd been curious about anal sex for a long time, but I couldn't get Connie, my wife, to go along with it. 'It's going to hurt too much,' she argued. And the only time I tried—just a little—sure enough, it seemed like there was no way my penis was going to fit in there. And yet I'd read, and even seen films, about supposedly normal women who could fit entire fists into their rectums without any ill effects. My wife was normal in all other physical respects, and my penis was about average size.

"Finally I read an article that made a lot of

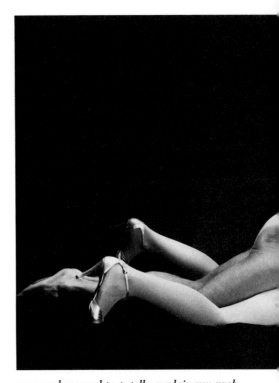

sense and seemed to totally explain my problem. It said that the reason most women couldn't have anal sex was because they thought it would hurt. They tensed their rectal muscles as a reflex precaution against the pain they believed was coming. This then became a self-fulfilling prophecy, because when a woman tenses her anal muscles, her anus actually does become too tight to accommodate a penis. The article went on to say that the way to overcome a woman's resistance to anal sex was to get her to relax. The method that made the most sense to me was described in the article as the gradient-step system. Simply put, it was up to the man to make his partner feel confident and comfortable with the idea of anal sex gradually, over a period of time.

"The night after I read the article, I made my first move. Every once in a while as we were making love, I toyed gently with Connie's anus. The next time we made love, I did a little more of the same thing. Gradually I worked up to putting a lubricated finger just inside her anus, then gently withdrawing it. Over a period of weeks, I put the finger more deeply inside Connie, and she never said a word. I always did

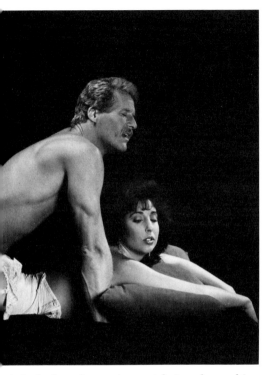

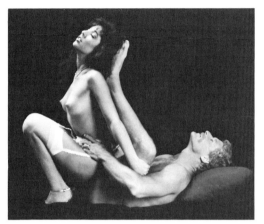

until finally we were going at it as wildly as we did when I was inside her vagina. After Connie adjusted to the unfamiliar—though not painful—feeling, she enjoyed the experience very much. In fact, she had two orgasms before I got out of her anus. Then I washed and dried myself with a soapy washcloth and towel I had remembered to put by the bed, and finished with a fantastic orgasm deep inside her vagina.

"Although anal sex has not become something Connie and I do every night, we toss it in every once in a while to add some variety.

The bottom line on anal sex is that it can be performed, and that it is not a perverted act. However, you and your partner must use common sense and mutual trust to make it a truly exciting variation of sexual pleasure.

it lovingly and never in a quick, 'sneak attack' fashion.

"Finally, one night after Connie and I had gone to a party and we were both feeling a little loose, I decided to make my move. We got into our usual position for rear entry, with Connie on her knees, her ass in the air, and me right behind her. Since I'd been gradually getting Connie to adjust to anal sex over a period of time, she didn't even flinch when I gently eased a lubricated finger into her anus. Deeper and deeper I put my finger into her anus. With my other hand, I was liberally lubricating my stiff cock.

"Finally the moment of truth arrived. I guided her ass into position and dabbed some extra lubricant around her anus. Slowly—and I can't emphasize this enough—I put my penis against her anus, then just barely pressed it inside. I felt Connie jump a little, but she was familiar with the sensation of having something in her anus, and she trusted me enough to know that I wasn't about to 'ram' something up inside her. When she tried to pull away, I gently guided her back into position. Very slowly, I was able to put my entire penis inside her, inch by inch,

> **IMPORTANT MEDICAL PRECAUTIONS**
> The rectal sphincter is extremely sensitive and should be stimulated with the utmost care. The rectum has a small supply of its own internal mucus, but it is not enough to ease insertion and properly lubricate intercourse. Apply a liberal amount of <u>water soluble</u> jelly to the anus before inserting anything. Due to the opposite chemical nature of the rectum and the vagina, do not insert anything (vibrator, penis, finger, etc.) into the vagina that has been in the rectum without carefully washing it.

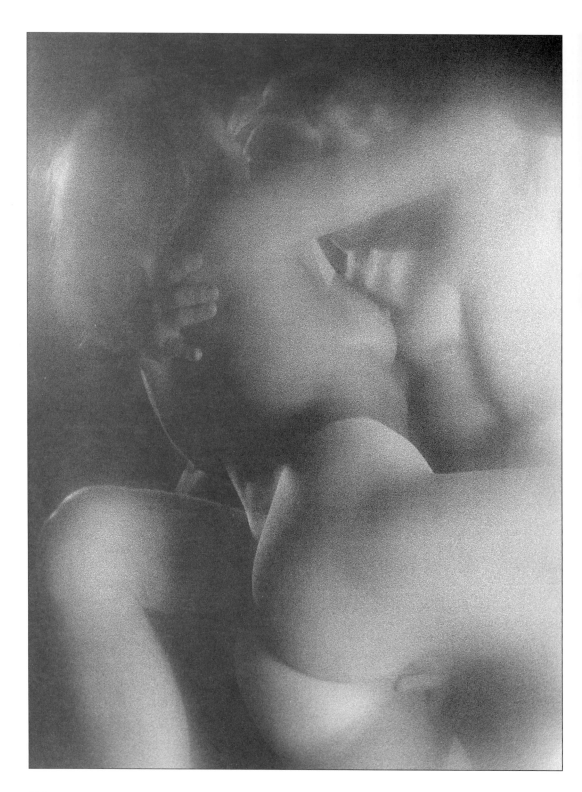

EROTIC EYE

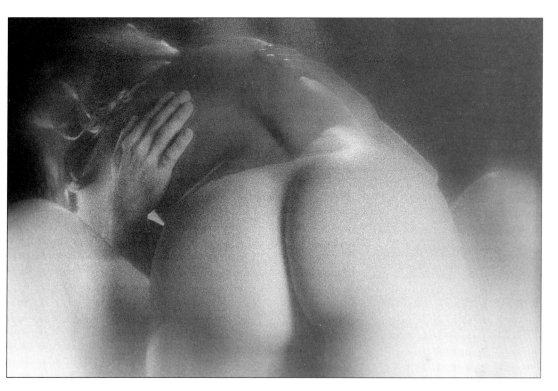

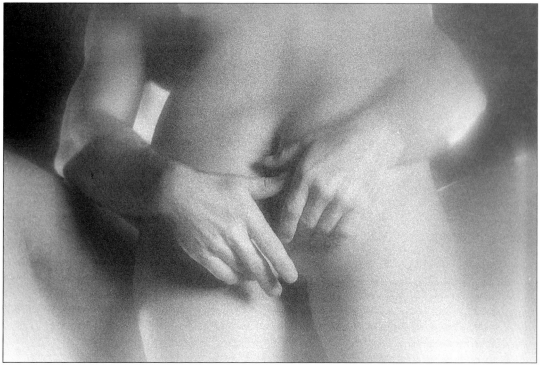

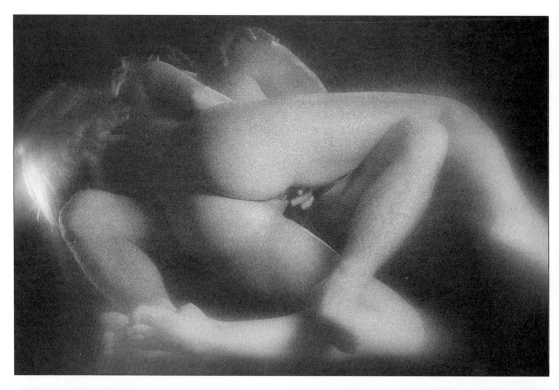

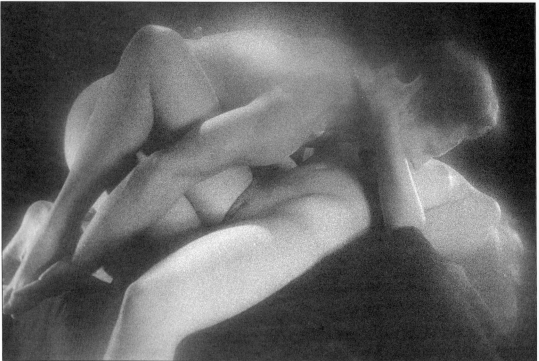

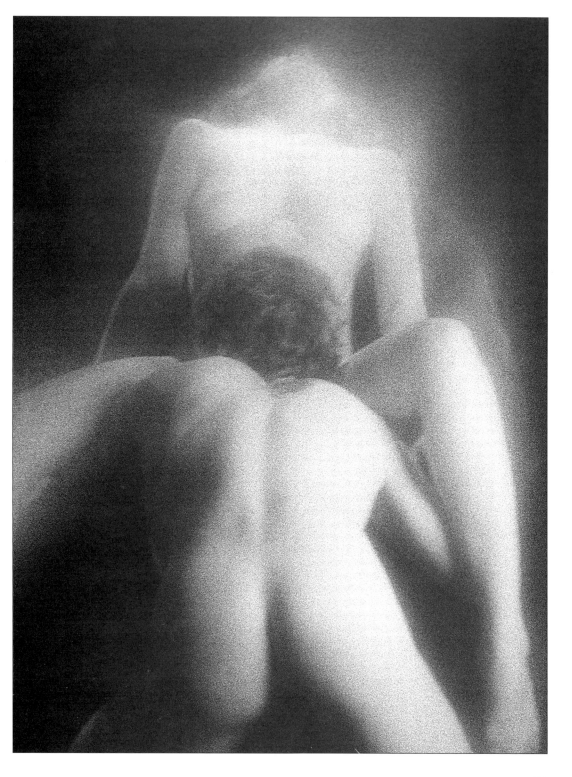

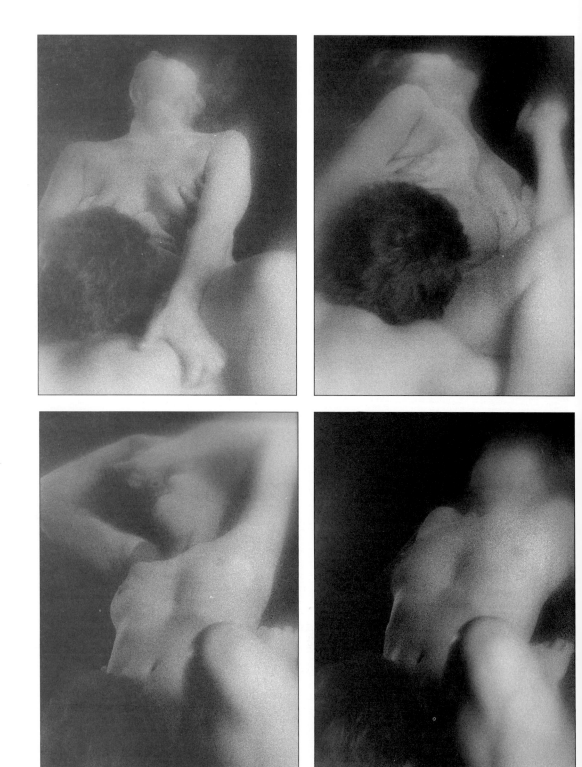

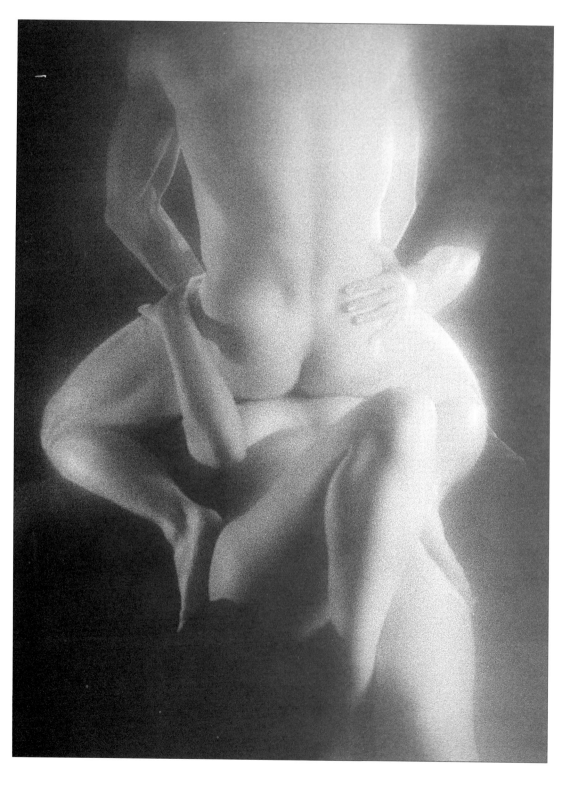

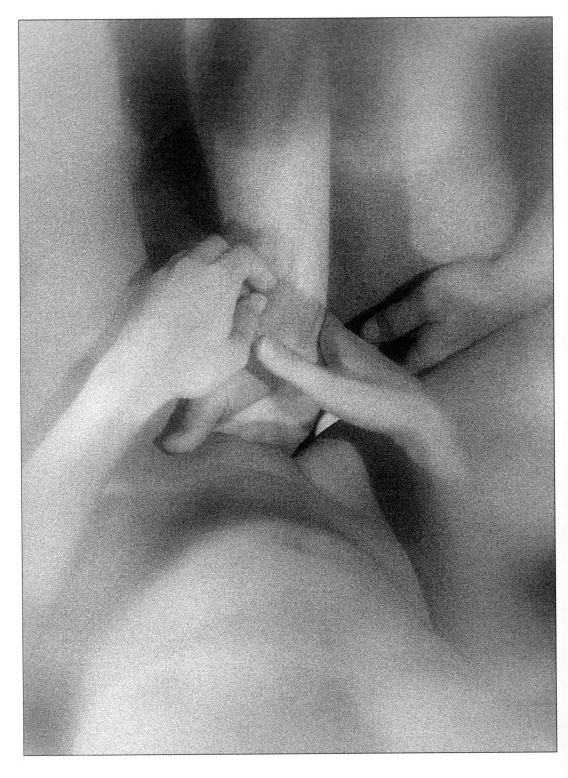

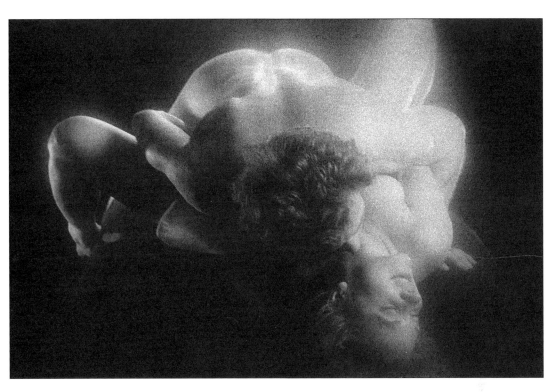

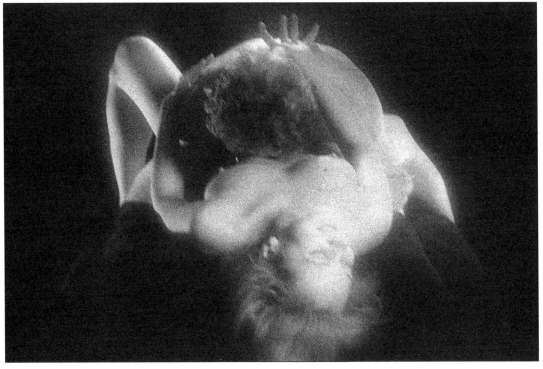

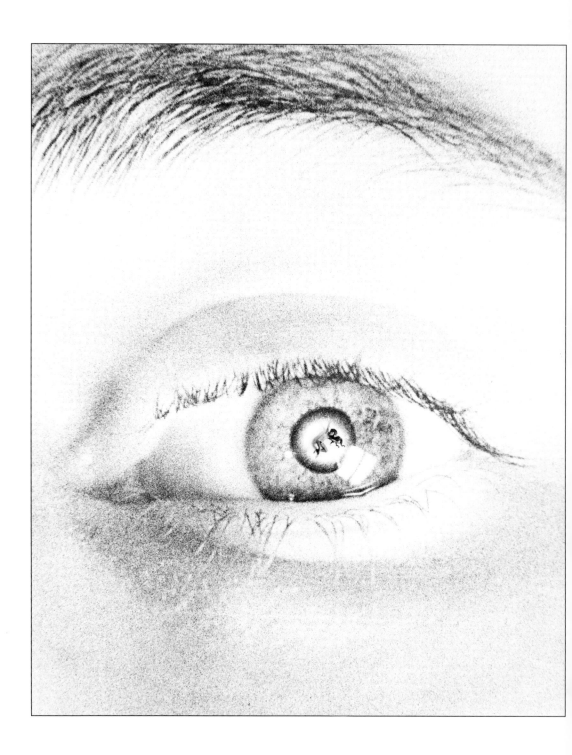

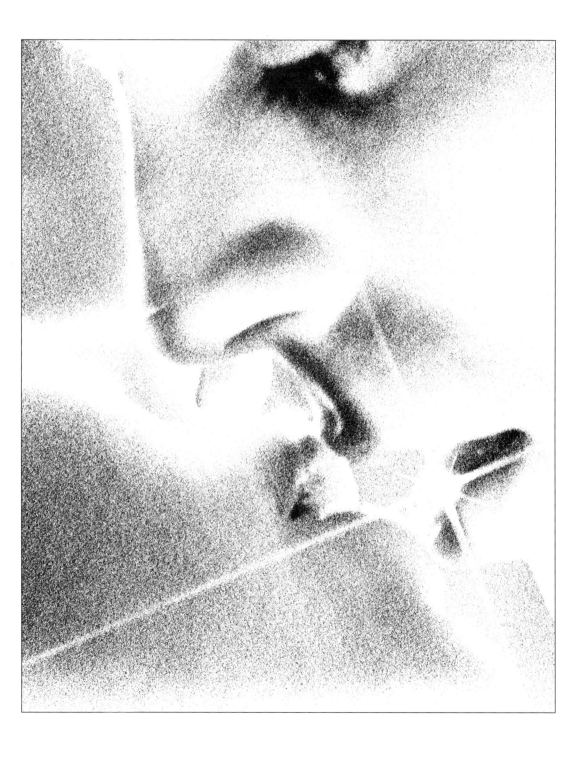

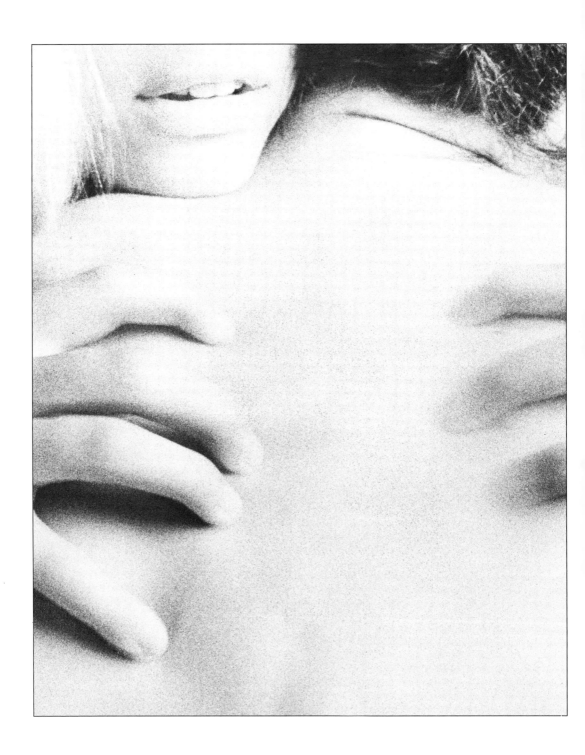

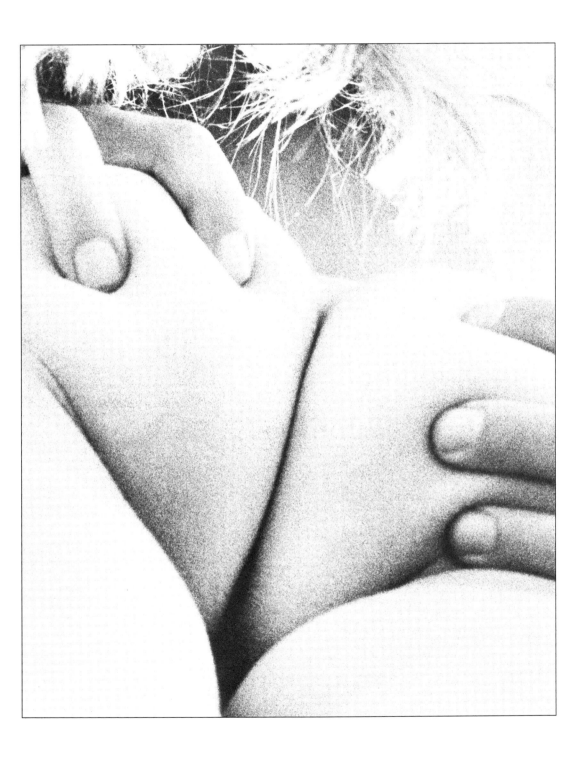

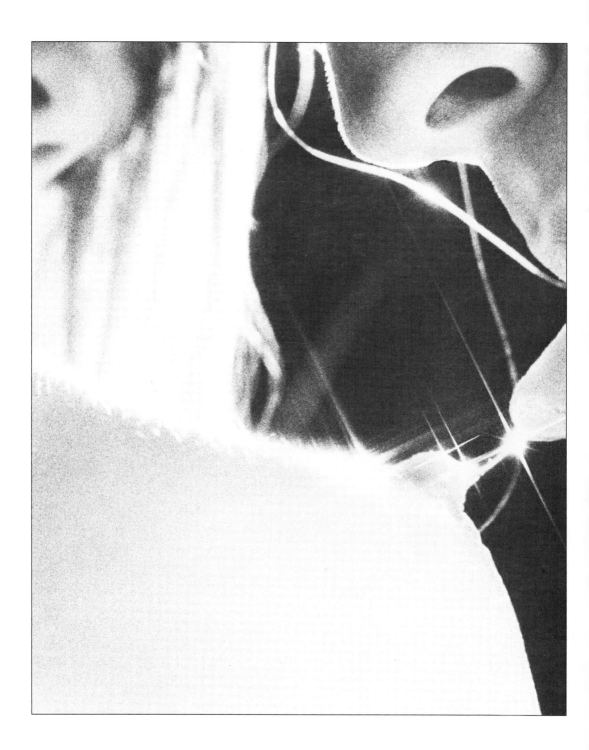

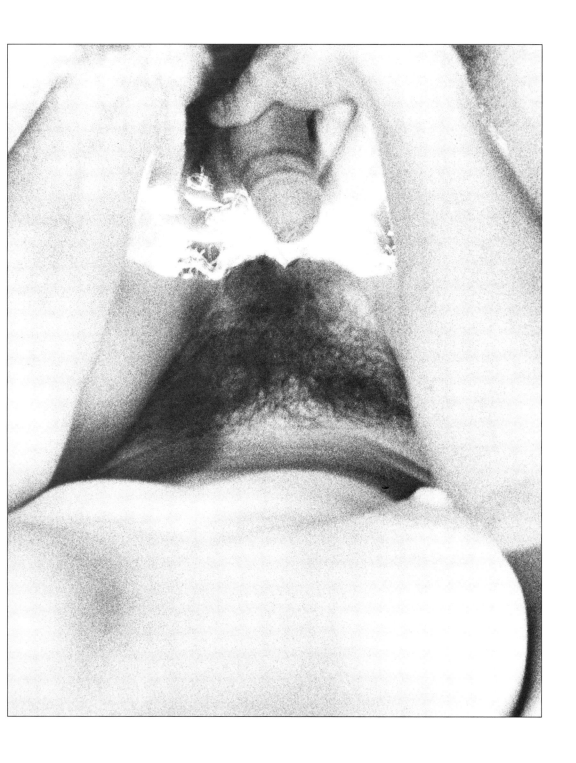

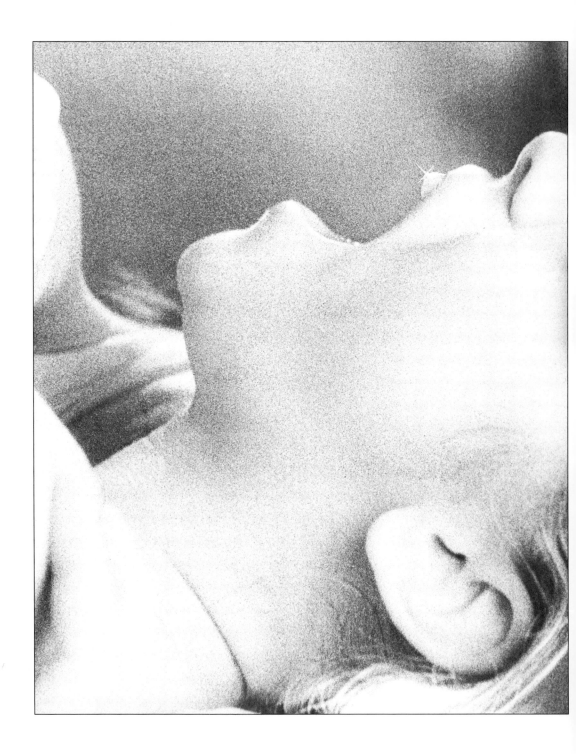

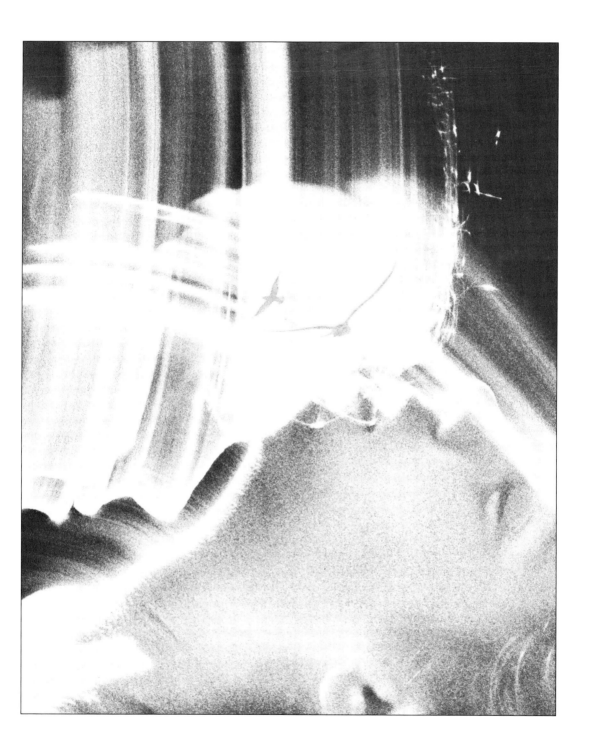

A·FINAL·THOUGHT

While I was writing this book, John, a good friend of mine, and I were tipping a few at a local watering hole and talking about—what else?—women.

The conversation naturally came around to this book. John was full of stories and "insight" regarding the various subjects contained herein. His exploits, if he can be believed—and I give him about a 75% believability rating—provided him ample grounds upon which to base his many opinions and recommendations. John has been a bachelor ever since I've known him— which is about seven years—and he's in his mid- to late thirties. He has had his share—and sometimes someone else's share—of women, having even lived with one during this period of time.

Around midnight, the conversation about the book turned to who could use it the most. John was sure that there wouldn't be anything in it he didn't already know. Then the name of a mutual friend came up—I'll call him Frank, though that's not his real name. John said that Frank could really use the book. Then John said a disturbing thing about Frank's girlfriend, Jane (also not her real name). He said, "I just can't see how a guy could make love to a woman like her. I mean, where *was* that girl when they were passing out looks?"

The remark really struck me hard. Though I agreed with John that Jane wasn't a real knockout, I'd never thought of her as a real bow-wow either. But the most interesting thing about John's remark was its contrast to a conversation I'd had only a few days earlier with Frank.

I was chatting about the book with Frank, and we were talking about women and sex. He and Jane have been together for about three years. He told me that even though he'd love to read my book, he was 100% satisfied with his sexual relationship with Jane and that, in fact, it had never been better.

Naturally, this intrigued me, so I asked him why.

"It's no mystery," he said evenly. "We love each other very, very much."

To be honest, on the surface that explanation sounded a little glib.

Sensing this in my vague response, he continued. "You know, Jane looks better to me today than ever. I used to think she was just okay looking, but now I really believe that she's beautiful. I mean, she really *looks* that way to me. We've been through a lot in the past few years: Jane's hospitalization, the loss of her father and my mother. Jane's a classy lady, a beautiful spirit, a kind, generous, and truly beautiful human being. She's taught me how to see a lot of what was in front of me most of my

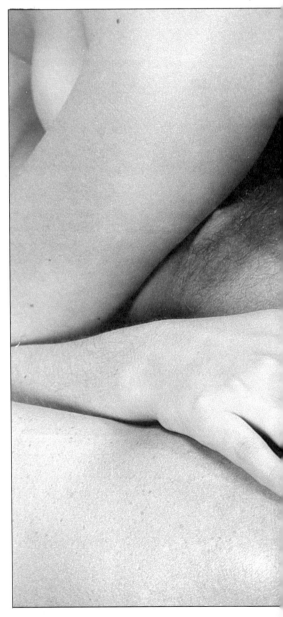

life, that I'd just never seen before. I really feel lucky that we've found each other.

"And getting back to what you originally asked me about—sex—it's the best sex I've ever had in my life. I realize that before I met Jane, I was just masturbating between someone's legs. I wasn't 'making love' with them, I was just grabbing hold of their bodies and using them to get myself off.

"I'm not saying that every time Jane and I make love it's the Fourth of July, but I *am* telling you that whenever I'm making love with Jane and I look into her eyes, I know there's someone there—really there—someone I care about, and someone who really cares about me."

Our ability to provide pleasure for, and derive pleasure from, people we care about is a truly wonderful gift. Share it with someone you love.

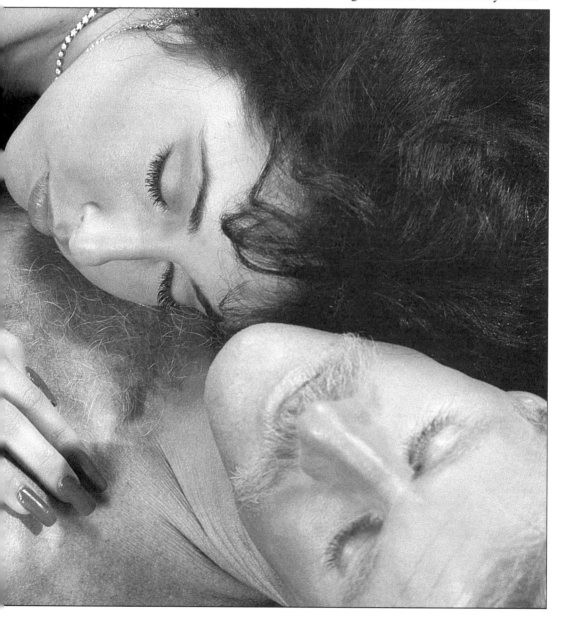

SAFE · SEX

BY KATHY KENNEDY

A popular television talk show hostess was quoted as saying, "It's hard enough to find a man you are attracted to, let alone putting him under an ultra-violet light or making him wear a condom—celibacy is sounding more and more reasonable." A recent newspaper article on being single advises all women to "avoid the sexy man who you know is promiscuous. He's dangerous."

We are assuming that you are an attractive woman or man, sexually active and that you are involved in a very exciting, sexual relationship. Maybe it's not totally exclusive, but it is getting close to that point. You have shared some titallating sexual experiences with your current lover and any playing around that is being done is usually out of town. Maybe an old lover might occasionally pass through town or a hot number from the office might become a one night stand . . . isn't that exclusive enough? We are a generation of people who have not worried about promiscuous sex until very recently. Sexually transmitted diseases like syphillis and gonorrhea were never considered fun, but let's face it, they aren't permanent or fatal, like herpes or AIDS.

We never had to worry about a virus that could be carried for five to seven years without so much as a warning rash. Now we are facing a virus that may attack our unborn children. Couples thinking about getting married have their entire lives flash before their eyes as they step up for a blood test and an AIDS screening. Remember that sweet boy you had a weekend with last year—didn't you always suspect that he was a bi-sexual? Then there was that wild blonde in New York; you spent an entire spring together, except when she would disappear for two and three days at a time . . . ever wonder if she used needles during her absences?

Everyone has a few of these stories in their not so distant past. Do we want to fess up to all of this with our present lover? Do brief encounters with homosexual ex-husbands or a swingers vacation taken five years ago have to be talked over? Well; yes. And no.

Of course, if you have been in a monogamous relationship for the last 10 years, and we do mean monogamous, where there is not a shred of doubt in your mind about who you have slept with, and you have no plans to expand your sexual horizons, then you personally have no need for this chapter. However, if you are like most of us, the information presented here could save your life.

Before a how-to session on sensual, safe sex can begin, there is a need to know if you have already been exposed to the AIDS virus. A simple, free, anonymous test is available and is effective at detecting exposure of up to two months prior to the test. We suggest these types of tests because they protect a person's identity, and that is very important.

Now we've been tested and we know we have never been exposed—it is our **most important responsibility** to keep it that way. We can now discuss how to stay clean while maintaining spontaneity, sensuality and the sense of sexual abandonment we have become accustomed to enjoying.

Relationships, like sexual activity, are as varied as the lovers involved. If you are involved in a strictly monogamous relationship and have been in it for seven to eight years, then sexually transmitted disease is not a personal issue for you. However, there are relationships where there is occasional promiscuous activity, and depending on the sobriety and sensibility of the partners, this could present a danger. Also there are relationships that are sexual, but not committed, where a couple may be terribly attracted to each other, have sex once or twice a week, but date and have sex with one or more different partners. This is definitely a threat. We must assume, in cases where other sexual partners are present, that they too will have other partners, and now we are dealing with more than the character of just the two lovers in question.

My lover is much younger than myself. We both have complete lives outside of our committed sexual relationship. Our commitment and intimacy is such that we have been able to discuss safe sex, other sexual partners, and our differing social directions. If he has sex with another woman, he uses a condom and I practice safe sex with any partners outside of our relationship. We both have been tested and know that we are not carrying the AIDS virus. This took a tremendous amount of understanding and coming to terms with our relationship and how we relate to the world outside of our

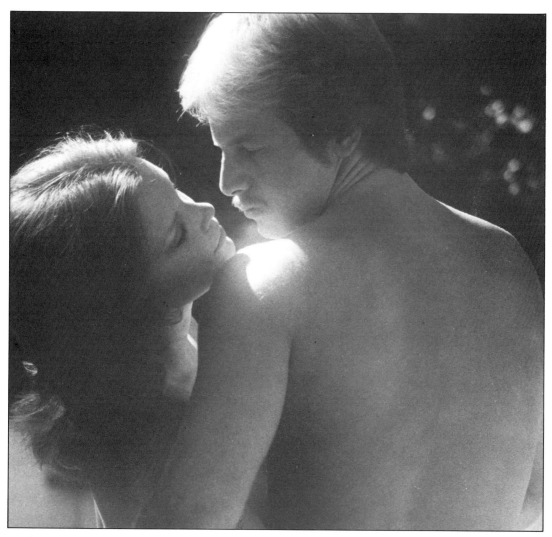

relationship. Ours is considered the primary relationship, marking all others as secondary. My lover would like to marry someday and have a family. My plans are to continue my education, become a doctor, raise my only child and never to marry again. In the meantime, we enjoy each other's company and have a wonderful sex life.

I have not found safe sex to be a problem. With the proper setting and confidence, I am convinced you can introduce medical precautions into your life and make them work. Talking about safe sex with someone you have just met or with someone with whom you are experiencing a first date, while you are both unsure of each other and nervous, or not even sure you are in fact going to have sex, is premature and awkward. I have discovered a simple solution to the problem and how to introduce safe sex effectively: I always end a date at my apartment and then at least I can be in control of logistics.

Once back at my place I fix drinks, turn on the music, lower the lights, and settle in for some romance. My date is a sexy man who finds me fascinating and desirable. I'm not going to turn on the ultra-violet light and try to find out if he has ever had sex with a man or an intravenous drug user, or if his girlfriend ever had a blood transfusion; at this point I wouldn't even ask him if he had herpes.

Kissing and fondling, maybe even a candle-light massage might be in order. This is a great way to check out genitalia for sores. Also, you can tell if a person is healthy or not by the glow of his skin. Massage is a hands-on way to feel a person's body and check for bruises, marks, or tracks. If I'm in question about a man's sexuality I concentrate on his buttocks to see how sensitive or aroused he might be when special attention is paid to the anal opening. This technique gives me an opportunity to get a good look at him without losing any of the specialness of the moment.

To safeguard against disease being spread orally, may I suggest that you do not brush your teeth before oral sex. The slightest tear or scratch to the gums could bring infected semen to blood. Do you swallow the semen is not a question I have ever been asked by a man, 'point blank.' That is one of our society's surprise perks. Considering the times and that this may be a first or second date with a would-be lover, I shouldn't be expected to swallow, and certainly he would not demand it. If the oral encounter goes on past foreplay, just stop when you sense your sex partner is ready to ejaculate. You can hand pump him and allow his semen to come on your stomach or breasts. It is a turn-on for a male to shower his cum on your breasts; don't underestimate the arousal factor of some of the simplest acts.

Now you are ready for coitus—this is when it becomes essential that this encounter is occurring at your place, and that you have cleverly hidden two or three condoms under the pillow. Look your lover right in the eyes, kiss him sensually and then with all the sex-positive attitude you can muster, open the condom and put it on his throbbing penis. Kiss him again and help him slide his protected erection into you. This could be the sexiest thing that has ever happened to him. Don't be surprised over his loving reaction when you are finished with this round. I suggest tucking away two or three condoms, because with this kind of sensual approach, there could be multiple lovemaking encounters in a single evening.

Now doesn't the scene I have just described make more romantic sense than two hours of nervous conversation about who has ever had sex with whom and how many times? Some-times my boyfriend and I practice one of the encounters I have just described because it is such a sexy thing to do. I have had men tell me that some women resent their use of condoms and feel as if a man is putting them down. Again, it's in the approach. If your date starts out moaning that he has to wear a "raincoat to take a shower" and he curses the day those "bad guys" brought us these dreaded diseases, then granted, safe sex will be viewed as a bad joke, and certainly a deterrent to the expression of physical love.

FROM A MALE'S PERSPECTIVE
The gentleman has a hot lady he just met in the bar of his hotel room. She is beautiful and needs a strong man to get her through the night. She has not mentioned safe sex, what she does for a living, or if any of her previous lovers have been bi-sexual men. She hasn't even told you if she is having her period. Take her to your room and make a steam bath out of the bathroom by turning on the hot water and sealing the room with a towel. Order up cheese, crackers and a few more drinks. Help her take her clothes off and let her know that you two are going to have a steam bath together. Women will gleefully take off their clothes if they are assured the sexual encounter is going to be delayed. There is a common female fear of removing their clothes and being jumped on immediately. Now you are both naked, the bright lights in the bathroom are on and it's time to inspect. Look at her body; look at it affectionately and with great passion. Now rub her shoulders, her back, her legs; massage her mound and **look at her.** You want to know where her clitoris is (for later of course) and what her outer lips look like and how her vagina feels and how sensitive the opening to her vagina is. All of this can be done slowly and with innocent curiosity, preparing both of you for a better-than-most first sexual encounter.

Now you can see if the woman of your dreams has crabs or sores, or is a woman for that matter. And she can know that you aren't laying on top of her with a pulsating, no-conscience penis. And, best of all, talking and touching in the steamy, bright lights of the hotel bathroom is an incredible turn-on. It has worked on me more than once.

You have talked, laughed, observed and hopefully touched your new lover's skin. You have looked into her eyes and you are both so turned-on you may not make it to the bed. Have your condoms stashed in the bathroom, so if you can't get to the bedroom for coitus, you are ready. Open the condom, kiss her, look into her eyes, take her hand and rub your penis with it. Help her help you put the rubber on. Tell her how beautiful she is and how you can't wait to feel your penis in her. This whole experience will be viewed by her and by you, not as a safety precaution or that you don't trust her, but as sharing, passionate foreplay. When the lovemaking is about to climax, tell her you want to come on her stomach or ask her if she wants you to come on her breasts. Talk about how you feel about her sexually; do not dwell on the topic of having to wear a condom to be safe.

Back to the primary relationship of the "almost" love of your life. If you both want to be extra safe, then by all means practice the same safe sex methods. However, if you feel that the commitment you share is trustworthy enough (and only the two of you can work that out) then feel free to indulge yourselves, because you have protected both partners by applying safe sex methods to your outside activities. All the health books, self-help and relationship manuals that I have read, say the one thing to guarantee a long, healthy life is a primary, committed relationship. Everyone needs someone in whom they can confide and someone who can be trusted to nurture them and their secrets. If nothing else, hopefully the recent open discussions of sexually transmitted diseases have given existing committed relationships a boost. Couples have commented that they feel it is better to risk a committed relationship than disease—not my favorite reason for wanting to be involved in trusting another human being, but certainly a rational attitude.

For my boyfriend and I to come to these kinds of terms required some long, and sometimes heated, discussions. We had to be totally honest with each other and candidly reveal what we enjoyed about spontaneous sex partners. We also discovered that the excitement lost after the first few months of a relationship isn't necessarily something lost, but actually something very 'special' found. Spending time with others with different sexual interests and trying to discover if they are high-risk people, has let us know more about the ramifications of a "one night stand" than just the thrill of the moment. Knowing a person a little better doesn't take away that excitement of first time sex, but actually keeps it in a better perspective. That beautiful blonde might make you hard at the thought of her, but is she as sensitive as your primary lover? And that dark, blue-eyed hunk may give drop-dead-head, but breakfast with him everyday might be a bore.

My partner and I have benefited from safe sex practices and I hope you and your mate will too. Whether you and your partner decide to use these techniques with each other—perhaps to keep either of you from getting something one of you already has, or perhaps you are not ready for complete trust—you can still enjoy sex and be safe.

There are certain sexual practices, like anal sex, though once enjoyed, that I would not indulge in again. But all the things that go along with sex that I really love are safe: music, soft lights, mellow conversation, good wine, touching, body rubbing, massage, gentle kissing and many more.

The local health department offers a few common sense techniques that will help you stay safe: shower before and after sex; have sex in your own home whenever possible; cut down on alcohol and drug consumption so your decisions about who you sleep with are more sound; never brush your teeth right before oral sex and if you do take semen in your mouth, wash it out immediately with an antiseptic (any 100 proof alcohol will do). Fist-fucking is extremely dangerous, even more so than anal sex—**avoid any sex act that might make you bleed.**

If you avoid high risk groups: bi- and gay men, intravenous drug users, hemophiliacs and people who have had massive blood transfusions, males of Caribbean descent and all those incredibly sexy gals and guys in every bar who have a reputation for whoring around or womanizing, you will probably not contract a sexually transmitted disease. Please do not stop pleasuring yourself or your lover. Do not pass up a chance for sexual happiness due to paranoia—do enjoy, do be sexy, do have fun, and practice sensual, safe sex.

G-SPOT POSITIONS

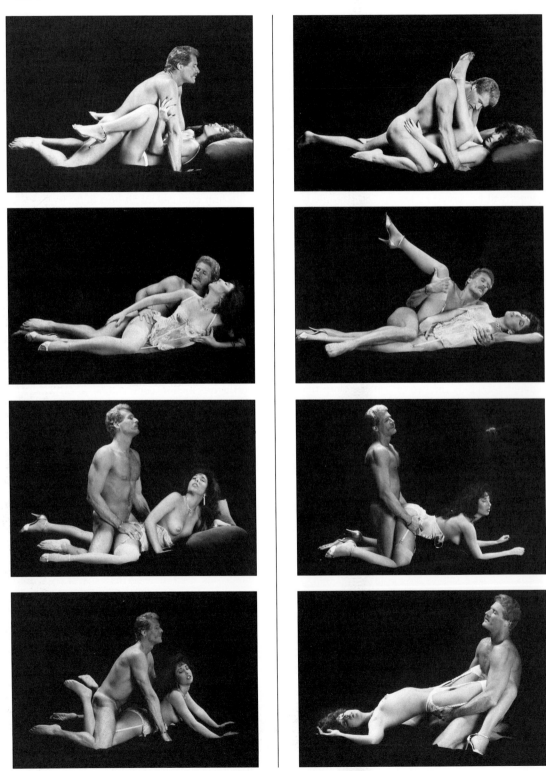